#1 BEST-SELLING AUTHOR

Dr Libby's

The Calorie Fallacy

Stop Dieting
Start Nourishing

DR LIBBY WEAVER

Disclaimer

The contents of this book are for information only and are intended to assist readers in identifying symptoms and conditions they may be experiencing. This book is not intended to be a substitute for obtaining proper medical advice and must not be relied upon in this way. Always consult a qualified doctor or health practitioner. The author and publisher do not accept responsibility for illness arising out of the failure to seek medical advice from a doctor. In the event that you use any of the information in this book for yourself or your family or friends, the author and the publisher assume no responsibility for your actions.

Published by Little Green Frog Publishing Ltd
www.littlegreenfrogpublishing.com

ISBN: 978-0-473-29237-9

For Dr Merv Garrett, with much gratitude for fostering
my independent thinking

Also by Dr Libby Weaver

Accidentally Overweight

Rushing Woman's Syndrome

Dr Libby's Real Food Chef, with Chef Cynthia Louise

Beauty From the Inside Out

Dr Libby's Real Food Kitchen, with Chef Cynthia Louise

Registered Reader

Congratulations on purchasing *The Calorie Fallacy*. The science and understanding of the impact that nutrition and lifestyle choices have on our bodies is constantly changing as colleagues in the research world continue to make breakthroughs.

By purchasing this book you qualify for our Registered Reader program. Our aim with this Registered Reader program is to ensure that we are able to keep you abreast of the latest developments in health and well-being, as well as provide you with a touch point to continue to motivate you to achieve the goals you desire for your health and body.

Please become a registered reader by visiting:
www.drlibby.com/registered-reader

Contents

*M*y mission is to educate and inspire, enhancing people's health and happiness, igniting a ripple effect that transforms the world.

cal·o·rie *noun*

a unit of heat used to indicate the amount of energy that foods will produce in the human body

plural **cal·o·ries**

1a: the amount of heat required at a pressure of one atmosphere to raise the temperature of one gram of water one degree Celsius that is equal to about 4.19 joules — abbreviation *cal* — called also *gram calorie, small calorie*

1b: the amount of heat required to raise the temperature of one kilogram of water one degree Celsius : 1000 gram calories or 3.968 Btu — abbreviation *Cal* — called also *large calorie*

2a: a unit equivalent to the large calorie expressing heat-producing or energy-producing value in food when oxidized in the body

2b: an amount of food having an energy-producing value of one large calorie

Origin of CALORIE

French *calorie,* from Latin *calor* heat, from *calēre* to be warm — more at lee

First Known Use: 1866

cal·o·rie *noun*

(*Medical Dictionary*)

plural **cal·o·ries**

Medical Definition of CALORIE

1a: a unit equivalent to the large calorie expressing heat-producing or energy-producing value in food when oxidized in the body

1b: an amount of food having an energy-producing value of one large calorie

calorie *noun*

(*Concise Encyclopedia*)

Unit of energy or heat. Various precise definitions are used for different purposes (physical chemistry measurements, engineering steam tables, and thermochemistry), but in all cases the calorie is about 4.2 joules, the amount of heat needed to raise the temperature of 1 g of water by 1°C (1.8°F) at normal atmospheric pressure. The calorie used by dietitians and food scientists and found on food labels is actually the kilocalorie (also called Calorie and abbreviated kcal or Cal), or 1,000 calories. It is a measure of the amount of heat energy or metabolic energy contained in the chemical bonds of a food.

Merriam-Webster's
Collegiate Dictionary

And this I believe: that the free, exploring mind of the individual human is the most valuable thing in the world. And this I would fight for: the freedom of the mind to take any direction it wishes, undirected.

John Steinbeck

Introduction

If you were with me when I was at university, you would have
seen me head out the door to go for a run, six out of seven days
a week — if not seven out of seven days — and usually for two
hours. I was healthy, happy, slim, and life was good. I would
run each day thinking I was doing so for fitness, which I was,
but in hindsight I can also see I was doing it to stay slim, as the
importance of burning calories had been drummed into me in
my earlier education.

But then I got a job running a health retreat and had to leave
home at 4.20 in the morning to arrive at work by 5.30am to
wake the guests. I loved the drive and the early morning air.
Sometimes I drove in silence; other times I listened to the radio
or to a cassette tape. By 6am at work I was teaching qigong, a
slow and gentle moving meditation during which you breathe
from your diaphragm. My next job for the day was to take the
guests who were either recovering from illness or injury, or
who may not have exercised for some time, on what was called
the "easy walk", 20 minutes over flat ground. I didn't break a
sweat, but rather enjoyed chatting to the guests and soaking
up the lovely scenery. My eating remained the same across
these periods of my life.

So, I had gone from being Little Miss Runner, burning
bucket-loads of calories, to Little Miss T'ai Chi, hardly burning
any at all. I had stopped running when I started my job, as I
was leaving for work in the dark and arriving home in the dark,
and I wasn't so obsessed that I was prepared to go running at
3am. I also noticed that on my two days off I missed qigong,
and so I would walk into the bush behind my house and find a
clearing in the early morning sunlight and do my practice for

30 minutes. I liked how it made me feel, even though I couldn't articulate any more precisely what that feeling was. I just knew I liked it.

Yet despite burning significantly fewer calories with my new daily routine, my clothes got looser and looser. This completely fried my brain, because, based on the way I had been educated, the precise opposite was supposed to happen.

It was this experience, coupled with what I was noticing more and more in some — not all — clients, and particularly in my female clients, that lead me to go back to my geeky biochemistry textbooks. The questions in my mind were: "What leads the human body to get the message that it needs to store fat?" and "What leads the human body to get the message that it needs to burn fat?" And I put the answers to those questions into my first book, *Accidentally Overweight*. The same information flavours this book, but this book is built around a different premise. I realized there was another story to bring to light, and that story fills these pages. That story is about the calorie equation and its inaccuracies, and what it omits to consider when it comes to what determines our body size and weight. It is also about the deprivation and fear that comes with the calorie equation approach, and how you miss out on life when food and a fear of food and body fat rule your thinking. It is about what happens when you know what to eat but no calorie equation, no diet, is ever sustainable and makes a lasting difference. You don't know why. All you know is that you feel like a failure because you can't stick to how you think you are supposed to eat, and you never feel like you do enough exercise. So you live with guilt and hopelessness most days of your life.

This book is about all of the parameters of the calorie equation, which was first published in 1918, and on which today's diet mentality is still based, and how it fails to factor in crucial elements of the modern world. For example, the calorie equation does not consider the metabolic consequences of modern-day food. It continues under the false belief that all that matters to body shape and size is your fat, protein, and carbohydrate (and alcohol) intake — the macronutrients from where you get your calories. But food for too many people today is no longer real. With each mouthful they get a host of different chemicals added to the food to enhance shelf-life or taste. And, as you will see throughout the pages of this book, this is one of the factors potentially messing with our ability to lose weight.

What I have learnt since my early qigong days has shaped not only my own health, but every ounce of work I have done since. Beforehand, if a client had told me that this had happened to them, that they had lost weight and body fat from burning fewer calories, in all honesty I am not sure I would have believed them. My education was so ingrained, and clearly said that if someone consistently ate more calories than they burned (you will see in a following section all of the things factored into this) they would gain weight. Yet I was burning far fewer calories, eating as much as I'd always eaten, and my clothes kept getting looser. And I was meeting more and more people who ate amazingly and moved regularly and they weren't losing weight. It all made me curious. It made me start asking questions. It made me not accept what I had been taught to be true for everyone. And it set me on a quest to free people from a relationship with food and their body based on the calorie equation, which was based on deprivation and fear. And that freedom is in these pages.

My Approach to Health

The way I approach people's health has three prongs to it: the biochemical, the nutritional and the emotional. This book is predominantly focused on the first two, although number three is touched on. The biochemical aspect of what I do explains how each body system works and the processes it undertakes, and the roles it plays. For example, I explain how and why we make stress hormones. The nutritional aspect of this approach explains the nutrients necessary for each body system to work optimally, and also covers the substances that can take away from the optimal functioning of a body system. The emotional prong helps people answer the question "Why do you do what you do when you know what you know?" For it is often not a lack of education that leads someone to polish off a packet of chocolate biscuits after dinner; it is biochemical or emotional, or both.

It's Time for a New Paradigm

I have witnessed countless people transform their bodies by relaxing and moving away from basing their food choices on the calorie equation. I have witnessed countless people go from eating a diet low in fat and high in complex carbohydrates, based on the food pyramid, and working hard doing five to seven cardiovascular gym workouts, in caloric deficit, and yet still constantly battling with their weight and experiencing weight fluctuations that they don't understand, and that the calorie equation cannot explain. I have witnessed them shift to a whole real-food diet, much higher in fat, do resistance training, gentle forms of yoga, stretching, qigong and/or walking; eating from 1200 to 2200 more calories per day than before, but not focusing on this, instead simply focusing on eating nourishing, nutrient-dense real whole foods. I have seen them lose weight, then stabilize their weight, and the results of any resistance work done in the gym is noticeable after one to two sessions, not months of hard slog. They never weigh themselves. Their clothes always fit. They have great energy and excellent health. Day after day. Year after year. It is truly transformational when you shift your focus from weight and calories to health and nutrition. It is, after all, nutrients that keep us alive.

> I have witnessed countless people transform their bodies by relaxing and moving away from basing their food choices on the calorie equation.

I have kept a diary since I was four years old. My dear mum gave me my first diary then, and I would write how many eggs

I collected from the chickens. Collecting the eggs was one of the highlights of my day. I still do it now when I visit my parents. I love it. But it started a practice that I have missed for only brief periods of time. It is where I have worked out many of my insights, including many about health. Here is one of those notes from a long time ago:

> Anyway, I just wanted to share this as I was quite surprised. I thought my carbs would be higher. The only "sugars" I get are from some rice milk I have sometimes, and vegies like potato, broccoli and cabbage, and lentils, so am sure that's a huge part of it. So even though a glucose/carb/sugar calorie is worth 4 and a fat calorie is worth 9, their metabolic effects were never considered when the HBE* was developed. And when food was only whole food and people ate simply, the metabolic effects were insignificant (and even though I hate the word toxicity), and this was partly because people weren't toxic from processed foods ... I know I'm raving on but there's something in this.

How many of us have been told that if we burn more calories than we eat, weight loss will be inevitable? How many of us have discovered that this century-old philosophy does not seem to apply to our body, no matter how hard we work, in this modern world?

In a world obsessed with calorie counting — as evidenced by the widespread listing of calories on food items and menus, and claims of the latest low-calorie miracle food, diet and exercise regime guaranteed to burn calories fast — we find ourselves instead watching the waistlines of the Western world continually expanding.

What if the foundation nutritional philosophy — that the calorie equation is the sole determinant of weight loss — is completely outdated, and in many cases wrong?

---

* HBE stands for the Harris–Benedict Equation, the mathematical equation used to calculate an individual's basal metabolic rate and their kilocalorie requirements.

I have written this book to help you stop dieting and start living. It is time to stop counting calories. If you want to count something, count nutrients. It is time for a new model of how to manage body shape and size. No longer are energy equations satisfactory in the information they provide. The concept that, so long as you eat fewer calories than you burn, you will lose weight, is well overdue for an update.

We will explore the fundamentals of weight loss that challenge the very core of weight-loss convention and dogma. I will share the journey that led me to piece together the biochemistry of sustainable weight loss, stemming from 14 years at university and 16 years in private practice, keenly observing how people do and do not respond to nutritional strategies.

Throughout these pages I will contest the assumption that you have to lose weight to be healthy, instead replacing it with a paradigm-shifting statement that in fact you have to be healthy to lose weight. This will transform how you view your body, and enhance your understanding of what your body requires to lose weight.

So for all of you who have been making an enormous effort and commitment to weight loss with little or no sustainable outcome, and for those who simply want to understand how to live happier, healthier lives, allowing your body to efficiently use body fat as a fuel, this book will arm you with the wisdom to stop dieting and depriving yourself, and instead to start thriving. Stop dieting and start nourishing yourself, and watch the transformation occur.

What's Ahead

Some people like detailed explanations of the mechanisms behind each of the concepts. I find it can make an enormous difference to change being sustained. For example, if I suggest you eat more fat from whole food sources, you won't necessarily do this until you see the extent of why and how this will make a difference for you. Or if I suggest you drink less caffeine, it will be much harder until you decide to do this for yourself with good reason, rather than just because you have been told to. However, I am also aware that some people just want the summary so they can get on with it. So both are in this book.

The Calorie Fallacy also contains case studies. All names and any identifying factors have been changed to ensure anonymity. Also, in some of the case studies there are test results included, while with others there are only symptoms. The treatment plan for each case study is not prescriptive; it is for educational purposes only, and I am not suggesting that what worked for the person described is appropriate for all people with that particular condition. I have included case studies so you can read about real people getting real results, and I hope this inspires and uplifts you, and guides you to a new freedom and nourishment with food and with life.

The most powerful force on Earth is the human soul on fire. Get fired up about treating yourself as the amazing human you are!

Dr Libby

Nutrients for Biochemical Reactions

Nutrients keep us alive, yet I feel most people don't hear enough about their importance. An adult's body is made up of about 50 trillion cells. That is a number that can go over our head with its enormity, as we tend to hear the word "trillion" on the news regularly, usually in reference to the US debt, and as a result it can seem like much smaller than it is. So I will use time as an example to demonstrate the enormity of 1 trillion, let alone 50. One million seconds ago was 12 days ago. One billion seconds ago was 32 years ago, but 1 trillion seconds ago was 32,000 years ago. Yet we are made up of about 50 trillion cells.

The Critical Role of Nutrients

Imagine you are made up of 50 trillion little tiny circles that all want to talk to each other, and the only way that they can communicate is when there are nutrients present. Imagine, then, what happens when people aren't getting adequate nutrients for some of the very basic processes, let alone for optimal health, as I believe is the case.

The cells of the body don't live forever. They are always in a cycle of replication, repair and death. Some cells turn over faster than others. For example, eye cells replicate quickly, whereas the bones do so slowly. Our whole outer layer of skin is replaced every 28 days! However, the health of the next generation of cells is dependent on the information they pick up on in their environment. And what's in their environment? Either nutrients or a lack of nutrients, one nutrient or many. There are also hormones at work — and at this point in the book, we will divide them into the categories of love and fear, for simplicity's sake — which are activated when we feel loving, appreciative feelings, and also when we feel fearful. The health and quality of each new cell is powerfully influenced by this information.

When I was doing my undergraduate studies in nutrition and dietetics, as well as during my PhD in biochemistry, I had the biochemical pathways of the human body mapped out on large pieces of paper, stuck to my bedroom walls. It was the only way I was ever going to learn them. When you see the body mapped out like this, you get a deep appreciation for the critical role nutrients play in life itself. Every second there are billions of biochemical reactions taking place. What that means is that substance X has to be turned into substance Y, and for that to occur perhaps you need magnesium and vitamin B_6. Without one or both of these nutrients the reaction can't occur efficiently, and so substance X accumulates and you miss out on substance Y. And maybe if substance X accumulates it behaves as a toxin, something your body will need to get rid of (more on toxins in the "Adipose Tissue" section later), and perhaps you need substance Y to sleep restoratively, or to create the hormones that allow you to feel happy, or for you to be able to access body fat and burn it as a fuel.

When you see the body mapped out like this, you don't just get a deep appreciation for the critical role nutrients play in our health, but you also get a deep appreciation for the absolute miracle that we are. If you knew who you truly are, you would be in awe of yourself. However, too few people live their lives in touch with that, and therefore don't treat themselves accordingly.

Your Role

Due to the incredible advances of Western medicine we are going to continue to live longer and longer. We are so fortunate to live in a time where there is such extraordinary emergency medicine available to us. Yet are we living too short and dying too long? It is an important question to ponder; for what I care about is the *quality* of that life. Today, as well as in the later part of your life, you still want to be able to bend over and do up your own shoelaces. Imagine what life would be like if you had to rely on someone else to do this? How would your once-independent self feel? You don't want this to happen because your tummy has grown too large for you to be able to reach your feet, and so you sit back now and wish you had changed the way you eat earlier. You don't want to not be able to reach your feet because you have led a sedentary lifestyle and now your spine is relatively inflexible and you can't bend to reach your feet. You don't want that to occur. And the ways you eat, drink, move, think, believe and perceive don't just impact how you feel, function and look today — they are going to influence how you feel, function and look in the future. And the power to change all of that is in your hands, and in *your* hands only. Let that empower you.

> The way you feed yourself is the most basic, most fundamental way you demonstrate care for yourself.

The way you feed yourself is the most basic, most fundamental way you demonstrate care for yourself. It is time to stop dieting and start nourishing. It is time to stop counting calories; if you need to count anything, count nutrients and ramp them up, and count synthetic substances and omit them. You will see why and how throughout the pages of this book. Remember, it is nutrients that keep us alive.

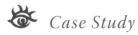 *Case Study*

Melissa's Story

Melissa, 46, was a classic calorie counter who said when she walked in that she could "quote the number of calories in a digestive biscuit." In other words, she knew how many calories were in many foods off the top of her head, she'd been so engrossed in that way of living for such a long time. She came to see me for weight loss and some insight into why her weight seemed to fluctuate despite her eating 1800 calories a day and never eating more than 2000 calories per day, "perfect for my caloric needs." She expressed adamantly that she never exceeded this. She just couldn't understand why, when she ate "so well", that her weight was never stable. Her frustration and sadness about this had been heightened just prior to her seeing me when her GP told her she was clinically classified as overweight and that she needed to lose weight.

When I took Melissa's diet history, it showed she ate:

Breakfast:
Bran flakes with skimmed milk
1 piece of wholemeal toast with a scraping of margarine
Morning tea:
Nothing

Lunch:
"Never more than a basic sandwich or a salad"

Melissa kept her calorie intake during the day to 800 calories so she could "allow herself a reasonable evening meal with my family".

Dinner:
Pasta or curry
2 glasses of wine
Drinks:
   "I drink endless cups of black tea and black coffee to keep hunger at bay."

Melissa said she felt "ratty" by the early evening and was

easily frustrated with family members. She also experienced headaches after eating, bloating and indigestion, and she said she felt constantly exhausted. She said her calorie counting went as far as disrupting eating out occasions, so much so that she tried to avoid socializing when food was involved. If she couldn't avoid a dinner (which was rare she said), she had worked out a way of messing her food up on her plate so the waitress and others at the table would think she had eaten some. She preferred to do this with a main course and eat her calories as a dessert.

Melissa's life had been taken over with her focus on food and avoiding calories, and she lived in a constant attempt of weight loss. She said it consumed all of her thoughts and had done since her late teens. There is no joy in living this way, nor is there great health, energy and vitality. Plus weight fluctuations and fluid retention are common with this way of eating. Melissa's diet was low on most nutrients, and most of her meals came out of packets and were highly processed, despite them being labelled as "low fat", for example. Yet, Melissa thought she was doing everything right.

I guided Melissa to shift her focus to her health and resolving the symptoms she had described. I asked her not to weigh herself, which she said she couldn't do, so we compromised and she weighed herself monthly. You have to be able to weigh yourself without judgment before you can weigh yourself out of curiosity, and I felt that would be a journey for Melissa. I guided her to eat a whole food diet, but she was initially concerned at the amount of fat, given that in her mind, it was so high in calories. However, after some more explanations of biochemistry and metabolic processes, like those in this book, Melissa started with her new way of living.

She joined me a few months later at one of my weekend events, and she immediately looked younger and leaner to my eyes. She also looked more relaxed and happier. It was as if her face had softened, not that I had thought it looked hard when I first met her. By the end of the weekend — where she obtained the whole big picture of the way the biochemical, the nutritional and the emotional aspects of health interact — she said she was thrilled to be on her new path of nourishing her body, mind and soul, and that she loved the results of living this way.

Too many people undervalue what they are,
and overvalue what they're not.

Malcolm Forbes

The Calorie Equation

This section contains an explanation of the energy equation, which at times may seem a little wordy. I hope not, but please persevere even if you find this section boring. I need you to understand what the calorie equation is so that the rest of the book makes sense. If you don't fully understand it all, please don't worry: I will make the points you need to be aware of very clear. Some of you will enjoy this, though. It is about calculating energy requirements.

To maintain physiologic functions, the human body continuously expends energy via what is known as *oxidative metabolism*, usually described simply as *metabolism*. This energy is used to maintain chemical and electrochemical gradients across cellular membranes, for the biosynthesis of macromolecules, including proteins, glycogen (glucose from carbohydrates), and triglycerides (fats), and for muscular contraction. Your heart is a muscle, for example, and beats about 100,000 times a day, but needs to be fuelled with energy in order to do so.

Another aspect of energy is lost as heat. Energy expended can be assessed by two different techniques: what are known as direct calorimetry and indirect calorimetry. This information can then be used to calculate energy needs. What are known as "energy equations" also provide energy (calorie) requirement calculations.

Direct and Indirect Calorimetry

The term *indirect calorimetry* refers to how the heat released by chemical processes within the body can be indirectly calculated from the rate of oxygen consumption, which is expressed as VO_2. For the information sponges among you, the main reason for the close relationship between energy metabolism and VO_2 is that the oxidative phosphorylation at the respiratory-chain level allows continuous synthesis of adenosine triphosphate (ATP). Put simply, the respiratory chain is also known as the electron transport chain, which consists of a spatially separated series of reactions in which electrons are transferred from a donor molecule to an acceptor molecule, and this drives energy production in the body. In this case a biochemist would refer to the energy generated as ATP.

The energy expended within the body to maintain electro-chemical gradients, support biosynthetic processes, and generate muscular contraction cannot be directly provided from nutrient oxidation. Almost all chemical processes requiring energy depend on ATP hydrolysis — hydrolysis being the breakdown of a compound due to a reaction with water. It is the rate of *ATP utilization* that determines the overall rate of substrate oxidation and therefore VO_2. And VO_2 can be measured using equipment shown in the following diagram.

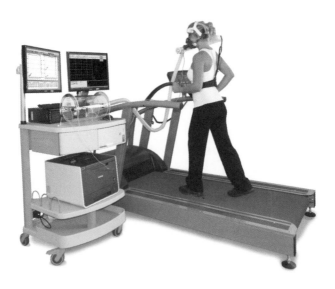

Source: http://en.wikipedia.org/wiki/VO2_max Wikipedia, 28 June 2014. Image by: Cosmed

Direct calorimetry consists of the measurement of the heat dissipated by the body by radiation, convection, conduction and evaporation. Under conditions of thermal equilibrium in a subject at rest and in post-absorptive conditions, heat production (measured by indirect calorimetry) is identical to heat dissipation (measured by direct calorimetry).

Put simply, the *basal metabolic rate* (BMR) can be calculated directly or indirectly through the measurements of key outputs. These are considered "direct measurements". The conditions required to obtain a precise BMR are very restrictive and require adherence to strict protocols. This method is, in most cases, generally impractical.

What is key to understand is that energy being utilized by the body can be calculated (some would suggest estimated), which I believe is highly applicable for athletes and in hospital settings. But its application to the general public is questionable, as primarily they don't have access to such machinery, and secondly what is expended changes due to the influence of many factors. It would therefore need to be recalculated regularly.

Equations

Another method to calculate calorie needs is to use equations that can calculate an individual's BMR. BMR is the largest component of *total energy expenditure* (TEE), usually ranging from 60% to 75%. The BMR is typically at the higher end of this range for sedentary people (70–75%) and at the lower end for athletes.

Harris–Benedict Equation

When I was at university I was taught that the way to calculate an individual's energy requirements was to use the Harris–Benedict Equation. It looks like this:

BMR calculation for men (metric)
BMR = 66.47 + (13.75 x weight in kilograms) + (5.003 x height in centimetres) − (6.755 x age in years)

BMR calculation for women (metric)
BMR = 655.1 + (9.563 x weight in kilograms) + (1.850 x height in centimetres) – (4.676 x age in years)

The Harris–Benedict Equation was revised in 1984 and became:

BMR calculation for men (metric)
BMR = 88.362 + (13.397 x weight in kilograms) + (4.799 x height in centimetres) – (5.677 x age in years)

BMR calculation for women (metric)
BMR = 447.593 + (9.247 x weight in kilograms) + (3.098 x height in centimetres) – (4.330 x age in years)

The scientific literature suggests that the revised version is believed to better calculate the energy needs of an obese individual.

Calculation of Caloric Requirements

Total caloric requirements equal the BMR multiplied by the sum of the stress and activity factors. Stress plus activity factors begin at 1.2 and are explained below.

Activity factors
The *activity factor* is used as a multiple to factor into the equation as a consideration for how much exercise a person does. Each category for the activity factor is listed below.

Sedentary: Little to no regular exercise — factor 1.2

Mild activity level: Intensive exercise for at least 20 minutes one to three times per week. This may include such things as bicycling, jogging, basketball, swimming, skating, etc. If you do not exercise regularly, but you maintain a busy lifestyle that requires you to walk frequently for long periods, you meet the requirements of this level — factor 1.375

Moderate activity level: Intensive exercise for at least

30 to 60 minutes three to four times per week. Any of the activities listed above will qualify — factor 1.55

Heavy (or Labour-intensive) activity level: Intensive exercise for 60 minutes or greater five to seven days per week (see sample activities above). Labour-intensive occupations also qualify for this level. Labour-intensive occupations include construction work (brick-laying, carpentry, general labor, etc.), also farming, landscape worker or similar occupations — factor 1.7

Extreme level: Exceedingly active and/or very demanding activities. Examples include: (1) an athlete with an almost unstoppable training schedule with multiple training sessions throughout the day; (2) a very demanding job, such as shovelling coal or working long hours on an assembly line. Generally, this level of activity is very difficult to achieve — factor 1.9

In a hospital setting, the activity factors are:

Bed rest — factor 1.2

Ambulatory — factor 1.3

Stress factors
Stress factors are based on whether an individual is injured or not. Along with the activity factor, this number (factor) is utilized in calculating total energy requirements. The stress factors are:

Surgery — factor 1.2

Trauma (severe, such as a motor vehicle accident) — factor 1.35

Head injury — factor 1.6

Sepsis — factor 1.6

Burns to less than 40% of total body surface area — factor 1.5

Burns to more than 40% of total body surface area — factor 2.1

Other than the activity factor and the stress factor (more accurately called the *injury factor* these days), nothing else is factored in as being an influence on caloric requirements and metabolism. I believe and have now witnessed too much evidence to suggest that this model needs updating, and the subsequent education of the public shifted dramatically as numerous other factors influence caloric requirements and utilization.

Other Measures and Issues

There are other equations also in use to calculate BMR and caloric needs. The Schofield Equation, first published in 1985, is one example. It omits height as a variable, and also considers males and females to have different activity factors, although they are still quite similar. But even this poses a question in my mind. Why have different activity factors for men and women? Women naturally have higher body-fat levels than men, even when both parties are super-fit. This is mostly due to oestrogen. And the world knows this. So why is a woman's oestrogen metabolism not considered to be an influencing factor on her caloric requirements and utilization? It is never talked about, and it needs to be, as you will see from the oestrogen and liver sections later in this book, particularly given the impact of oestrogen-mimicking substances in the environment that enter our bodies.

Again, there is also the issue of external environmental issues. For example, the Harris–Benedict Equation was first developed in 1918, just as World War I was ending. Consider how life was likely to have been then. To say that life has changed since then would be the understatement of the century.

Basal Metabolic Rate

The *basal metabolic rate* (BMR) is the amount of energy required to maintain the body's normal metabolic activity, such as respiration, maintenance of body temperature (thermogenesis), and digestion. Specifically, it is the amount of energy required at rest with no additional activity. The energy consumed is sufficient only for the functioning of the vital organs, such as the heart, lungs, nervous system, kidneys, liver, digestive system, sex organs, muscles and skin.

Science suggests that BMR generally deceases with age or if there is a decline in lean body mass. However, I postulate that BMR need not decline, certainly not significantly, due to age if regular strength training is undertaken to prevent the loss of lean and skeletal muscle. Activities that tend to increase lean tissue (muscle mass), including strength training and yoga, will also increase BMR. Aerobic activities, such as running and aerobic-based gym classes, may improve endurance but will have little effect on BMR, other than a brief, minor increase in the initial post-exercise state. You want to build muscle to improve BMR.

There is some literature reporting that stress, illness, hormone levels — they usually cite the thyroid — and environmental factors, such as temperature and altitude, may affect BMR. However, this is simply reported and is not factored into any of the equations used to advise people. Nor is any consideration given to the impact of other substances (toxins) that are stored in the fatty tissue of the body and their metabolic impact. Not that long ago in human history, if body fat was stored, it was more likely to have been just that — fat. However, as you will see in coming sections, the fatty tissues of the body can be storage houses for fat-soluble toxins from dietary and environmental sources, and no one has factored in the impact of this on metabolism, among numerous other factors which are the result of the world we live in.

Lean tissue requires significantly more energy to maintain due to its increased level of metabolic activity compared to fat cells. As a result, the fatty tissues of the body require very little energy to maintain, and have very little influence on the BMR. Hence, the greater the lean body mass, the higher the BMR.

Total Energy Expenditure

Science then teaches that the baseline BMR can be used along with an activity factor (outlined above) and a stress factor (referring to injuries such as burns or fractures and certain diseased states) to calculate an individual's daily caloric needs, referred to as *total energy expenditure* (TEE). This is expressed as kilocalories per day, which is often simplified to calories per day. The metric way to measure and describe calories is kilojoules, in the same way that distance can be measured empirically as miles and metrically as kilometres.

The TEE — the amount of calories needed per day — is composed of three primary factors: the BMR, the thermic effect of food, and physical activity.

Thermic Effect of Food

The expression *thermic effect of food* (TEF) is used to describe the energy expended by our bodies in order to consume (bite, chew and swallow) and process (digest, transport, metabolize and store) food. The TEF is calculated as the total number of calories consumed per day multiplied by 0.1. For example, if someone eats 2000 calories per day, TEF = 2000 x 0.1 = 200 calories per day.

However, even within that concept there are variables, as the thermic effect of protein is greater than that of carbohydrates and fats.

Shortcomings

All of the above equation work was ground-breaking in its day, and I readily acknowledge the contribution this work has made to our understanding of human physiology, its application in a hospital and critical-care setting and for athletes. I can see, and know first-hand working as a dietician in the emergency department of a hospital, that it was designed to save lives, and in that setting it does.

Where the problems lie are:

⁂ in the extrapolation of the data that the calorie equations offer to the general public

⁂ the restrictive, deprivation mindset that the calorie equations drive in those who adopt it (the majority of female clients I have worked with over the past 16 years), and that this deprivation is not sustainable

⁂ that it leads too many people to believe that they have to be constantly on a diet, living again with deprivation and often shame, from which you only end up deprived and ashamed

⁂ that it sets the majority of people up for a life of deprivation when they aren't following their low-calorie plan, or feeling guilty if they perceive they have eaten too much or exercised too little

⁂ that it can lead body- or weight-conscious people to restrict calories too much so that their metabolic rate slows (the point at which this happens will be different for everyone)

⁂ that it does not consider that the food supply has changed significantly since 1918 when the HBE was first published (and the 1984 revised version does not consider the change in food supply either)

⁂ that it does not consider the stress (true stress, not injury) and the stress hormone production of modern life via caffeine consumption and the perceptions of pressure and urgency

⁂ that it does not consider the impact of concentrated (refined) carbohydrates — both sugars and starches — on metabolism via insulin and also its subsequent blocking of leptin, an appetite regulator

⁂ that it does not factor in fat accumulation in the liver from alcohol consumption and a diet high in processed foods and drinks, and the impact of this on metabolism

⁂ that it does not consider the impact of the increase in oestrogen-like compounds in the food chain and environment, and their impact on metabolism

⁂ that it does not consider the impact of adrenalin or cortisol and their differing impacts on metabolism — given the acute and chronic stress experienced by too many people today, this is a major oversight

- that it does not consider that science has now shown that the bacteria inhabiting the large intestine can influence what calories are worth

- that it does not consider the impact of sub-optimal (or diseased) thyroid function, a major oversight given the significant rise in autoimmune thyroid conditions

- that it does not consider the impact of constant upper-thoracic breathing, instead of diaphragmatic breathing, and the impact of how an individual's natural way of breathing on a daily basis influences the body's fuel utilization via the autonomic nervous system (ANS)

- that it does not get to the heart of the matter if someone emotionally overeats

- that it does nothing to address why, if you see and feel your clothes getting tighter and you don't like it or you feel uncomfortable, you do nothing about it — why doesn't your self-care kick in?

In other words, the calorie equation fails to consider the bigger picture, physically, environmentally and emotionally, based on the world in which we now live. It is time for an update, as the foundation nutritional philosophy — that the calorie equation is the sole determinant of weight loss — is completely outdated. And it is time to thoroughly explore and start conversations in the street and in the research laboratories about the fundamentals of weight loss, and challenge the very core of weight-loss convention and dogma. It is time to stop dieting and start nourishing.

Diet History

The HBE was first published before there was a focus on low-fat foods, and before the advent of so many processed and highly refined foods. When the HBE was created, people ate mostly real food. Therefore, the metabolic consequences of carbohydrates, fats and proteins were straightforward, and they were worth their caloric value. However, now people often obtain their carbohydrates, fats and proteins mixed in with substances that the body has never been exposed to before, and potentially has no equipment (ie, digestive enzymes) to break down. Now, we get concentrated forms of carbohydrates and poor-quality fats in processed foods that in no way resemble the way the original foods were in Nature. In the not-so-distant past, if you went on a low-calorie diet it would only have been made up of fresh food, plenty of high-water vegetables, and some fruit and other whole foods. But now, if you eat packet low-calorie foods, they are low in calories because they are often made from non-food ingredients and chemicals, adding to what I will refer to in later sections as the "toxicity factor". This is a sure-fire road to poor health and, potentially, weight gain — and it is not an excess of calories driving that.

Too many processed foods also interrupt the regulatory cycles in the body that help us stop eating when we have had enough. The interference of high circulating insulin levels on leptin is one such example.

The Low-fat Era

I was educated at university when it was the "low-fat, high-complex-carbohydrate" era. Pasta was therefore considered to be a great food because it met these criteria. This made no sense to my brain, as it is low in nutritional value and looked nothing like the food from which is was derived. However, it was during the low-fat era that the waistlines of the Western world expanded like never before. There were now, among many other changes, fast-food outlets on every second corner in major cities, and often both parents were now working, changing how evening meals were prepared.

Instead of addressing the time-poor factor that was invading most people's lives, the powers that be sat back and proclaimed that it must be the carbohydrates making everyone fat, so roll on the high-protein, low-carb era we are now part of. For those of you who have been around long enough, you will recall that nutrition information moves in about 30-year cycles, and will continue to do so. During the low-fat era, the food industry responded to (or led?) the public's desire for low-fat options of their favourite foods. Where once there was just an ordinary apple pie in the frozen section of the supermarket, there was now a low-fat version on offer right beside it. If you were a health-conscious citizen at that time, you bought the low-fat apple pie.

However, when a food manufacturer removes most of the fat from a recipe, they leave a great big gaping hole. You can guess what they filled it up with, given that the people who were likely buying these foods had made a priority of how low the grams of fat on the nutrition panel were, and were only checking these. The manufacturers filled up the gap with refined sugar. But if you had been eating an ordinary apple pie and now you bought the low-fat one, and when you ate it, it was sickly sweet, you would have worked out what was going on. So to mask the increase in sweetness, they added salt, as salt masks sweetness in cooking. Therefore, if you followed low-fat dietary principles through this period and you included packaged foods in your diet, you ate more sugar and more salt than ever before in the entirety of human history. Yet you believed you were doing something supportive for your health.

It is important to be able to decipher nutrition information from food marketing. The way to not get caught up in food fads is to remember that, when it comes to food, Nature gets it right, and it is potentially human intervention that can get it so very wrong.

The Influence of How You Breathe

The science is very clear that the way you breathe communicates information from the environment to your ANS. But in modern times, when short, shallow (ie, thoracic) breaths are more likely to be a response to the caffeine you have consumed over the morning and/or your perception of pressure in your day, than to a woolly mammoth attack, the subsequent production of adrenalin, the mobilization of glucose, the inflammation, the interference in the anti-anxiety, antidepressant action of progesterone, the insulin, the fat storage messages, from that scenario *alone* is enough to alter your energy requirements. And for too many people, this is how they now live every day. I have included more about each of these topics in the coming pages.

The adverse health effects of poor breathing therefore need to be acknowledged, addressed and included in the action plan for improving health and body fat loss.

A New Paradigm

Therefore, I propose that it is time to be done with the calorie equation as a way of educating the public about how to eat. It is time to stop dieting and start nourishing. It is time to stop counting calories. If you need to count anything, count nutrients and increase them. Count synthetic chemicals and decrease them. Eat real food. Eat fat from whole food sources. Eat carbs from real food sources. It is easy to eat protein from real food sources; those sources have been played with much less than the carbs and the fats on the supermarket shelves.

Change your mentality: change the way you approach how you feed yourself to a focus on your health, not your weight. Positive not negative. A focus on what you can eat, not what you are not "permitted" to eat. Do not let it take a health crisis to remind you of what you already know: that without your health, you have nothing. Listen to your body. When you stop eating processed foods that interfere with your body's natural rhythms and signals, you will get back in touch with what your body, not your tastebuds, wants. You will learn to trust yourself again. You have your own inner doctor. Allow yourself to tune into her. Make your health a priority, and watch your health and body transform, and, just as wonderfully, free yourself from a life lived in the fear of weight gain, calorie counting, deprivation and never feeling good enough.

The calorie equation doesn't factor in what leads someone to over-eat. What it is that prevents us from doing something about a growing waistline when we notice our clothes are getting tighter or if we notice feelings of discomfort. The avoidance of emotional pain is the answer, and the calorie approach to health goes nowhere in addressing this. Look out for a deeper understanding of this in later sections of this book.

A Curious Experiment

Up until the time I wrote this book, I hadn't analyzed my caloric intake since 1999. So I used software to calculate my caloric intake and HBE needs from Australian and New Zealand food tables. Based on the HBE, I need 1812 calories for weight maintenance, and to lose weight it suggested I eat 1582 calories per day. I eat *on average* 2500 calories per day and my body rarely changes. Of that, 50% of my calories are coming from fat, 25% from carbohydrates, and 25% from protein. I am not suggesting you eat this way, as everyone is different, and I certainly haven't always eaten this way. It is what nourishes me now. I feed my body what it wants, and I have witnessed this change over time. It is just that I trust my body. I don't doubt it; I don't believe it has ulterior motives. It knows better than me, and I simply share this with you to show you an example of a discrepancy in a number that an equation generates, that many people take as gospel, to how someone with a very stable body size eats. I hypothesize, however, that if I ate 2500 calories of poor-quality, processed, highly refined foods, my body size would most likely increase. And that has nothing to do with calories and everything to do with the quality and wholeness of the foods, as well as the non-food ingredients (that I'm not eating) not interfering with detoxification processes.

Starting the Transition Away From Counting Calories

When I am asked for my number one health tip, my answer surprises people as it is has nothing to do with food. It is to diaphragmatically breathe. Consider this. The way we are created, we live for the shortest time without oxygen. Next comes water, and thirdly comes food. How you breathe plays a significant role in the information your body picks up on about what must be occurring in your environment. This is explained in detail in the section discussing the autonomic nervous system. But this is why diaphragmatic breathing is at the top of the following list, which is designed to help you begin your journey away from counting calories and towards vibrant health. Some of the reasons why I am suggesting these rituals be embraced are listed, too.

✱ *Breathe from the diaphragm:* Long, slow breathing communicates to the body that you are safe via the ANS, and you use body fat as a fuel effectively when the body knows it is safe.

✱ *Drink water, rarely anything else:* Hydration is critical to life, but also to the effective detoxification, filtration and elimination work done by the body.

✱ *Eat real food:* Your body has the enzymes to break this down, thus providing your cells with the nutrients they need for optimal health and function.

✱ *Build muscle:* This increases metabolic rate, improves insulin sensitivity, and improves blood glucose management.

✱ *Stretch:* Fascia is the specialized connective tissue layer surrounding muscles, bones and joints, giving structure to the body. It aids muscle movement, but also provides a passageway for nerves and blood vessels, and hence the exchange of nutrients, waste and energy. Therefore, flexibility is a conduit to good energy, hormonal function and detoxification. If the cells aren't receiving the nutrients they need, or aren't able to mobilize waste away from themselves efficiently, this too can cause stress and inflammation within the body, interfering with weight loss.

✱ *Adopt restorative practices:* Practices such as restorative yoga and qigong are excellent for parasympathetic nervous system (PNS) activation.

✱ *Sleep:* Get eight hours' sleep per night, and do your best to get two of those before midnight for hormonal balance and appetite regulation.

✤ *Reduce alcohol consumption:* Only drink alcohol on super-special occasions, to support efficient detoxification processes and hormonal balance.

✤ *Swap coffee for green tea or herbal tea:* Unless you are naturally very calm and/or don't have many demands on your time, caffeine-reduction will support an appropriate stress response.

✤ *Don't eat refined flours or sugars, artificial sweeteners, colouring, flavours or preservatives:* Doing so will help avoid the development of a fatty liver. (This might go without saying under the "eat real food" point, but I want to make it clear.)

✤ *Focus on health not weight:* This shift in focus will help give you great energy, vitality, happiness and freedom, as well as optimal health.

If all of that overwhelms you, begin by choosing one of those factors to focus on and incorporate additional new habits as you feel ready. You may choose to only focus on eating more real food, for example. You will certainly see why this is of such importance throughout the pages of this book.

This is not a book about rules or perfection, for they alone are not healthy. It is about holding a high standard for yourself and what you allow into your body, for as I mentioned earlier, if you knew who you really are, you would be in awe of yourself and you would treat yourself accordingly. I believe that the way we feed ourselves is our most basic form of self-care. It is what you do every day that impacts on your health, not what you do sometimes. It is how you *consistently* live that matters, and how you eat, drink, move, think, breathe, believe and perceive all impact on your well-being. It is time for the dawning of a new era in how people approach their level of self-care. And that has nothing to do with calories.

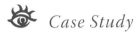 *Case Study*

Juliette's Story

Juliette was 27 years old when she sought my advice, as she was confused about why she couldn't lose weight despite "doing everything right". When taking her diet history, it was clear that she ate well most days of the week, only eating foods that didn't really serve her health on a weekend day if she had been out drinking alcohol the night before. Juliette did this on average once a month. She said she had had "weird eating habits" for a period when she was at university, and was quite body-conscious. She said she had exercised religiously at uni but had lived on cheap food, although she watched her calories very closely and said it was rare for her to ever eat more than 1700 calories a day.

Now, as a working woman, Juliette still counted her calories, and as a result ate very little fat, except for a quarter of an avocado on her salad for lunch, and the tablespoon of olive oil she "allowed" herself for cooking dinner. She occasionally ate nuts for afternoon tea, but always stressed about it, as she knew they contained fat and therefore had more calories than her usual few pieces of carrot or nothing.

Course of action
I explained to Juliette about all of the factors that can influence whether the human body gets the message to store fat or burn it, and I asked her to relax her calorie concepts and trial a new way of eating, which included eating only real food, and which had more fat from whole food sources. She said she felt nervous about doing this, but was nonetheless keen to give it a try, as she was sick of her body not responding to exercise the way she thought it ought to, and she was sick of worrying about it all so much.

Based on her age, weight and activity, we calculated that her requirements were close to 2000 calories per day. I only did this to demonstrate to Juliette that counting calories didn't serve her.

Outcome

As an experiment, Juliette still counted her calories as she started the new way of eating that we created. She ate an average of 2700 calories per day, and said that within a month she could finally see results from her weights sessions. The macronutrient breakdown had 48% of her calories coming from fat, 22% from protein, and 30% from carbohydrates.

My sense is that if she had eaten 2700 calories of processed food, even with the same macronutrient breakdown, the results would not be as substantial as they were. I also believe that if she had eaten 2700 calories and her macronutrient breakdown was higher in carbohydrates or excessively high in protein, the results also would not have been as great, due to the potential insulin response from the carbohydrates and the ammonia generation from the protein, and the subsequent load on the liver and kidneys long-term. I couldn't test this, as she (and rightly so) didn't want to change what she was doing, as she felt so good and was finally getting the results she wanted.

Another reason I believe this is so is that, prior to the dietary changes, she was eating just under 2000 calories per day and not getting the results. I don't actually count calories for clients, unless they are curious and want to experiment as Juliette did. She was now energized, nourished and living a life she loves and with no focus on weight, she lost weight.

Each morning upon waking, get in touch with what a gift life is:
to breathe, to move, to wonder, to love, to soak up.

Dr Libby

Fat Cells and Toxicity

We store energy in our body for later, in case we miss a meal or a famine strikes, so that we will have enough fuel to support the inner workings of the body that keep us alive. We store calories that weren't used straight away in the form of glycogen, which is stored glucose, fat and proteins. Proteins, when needed, can be broken down into amino acids and converted into glucose to be used as fuel. A person weighing 70 kilograms will store about 2500 calories as glycogen and about 130,000 calories as fat, which I will discuss in relation to sugar cravings in another section.

The fat we store in our body is not, however, just fuel for later. It fulfils many roles. Adipose tissue — fat cells — acts as an endocrine gland, which is a gland that secretes hormones. In the case of our fats cells, they secrete oestrogen in both men and women. And as you will see in another section, oestrogen itself is a fat-storage hormone, so the more fat cells we have and the larger they are, the more they make a hormone that signals fat storage, adding to the oestrogen being produced. One of many vicious cycles that needs to be interrupted for weight loss to occur.

An additional function of body fat is that it is a storage house for what I call "problematic substances". I could refer to them as "toxins", but that is a term that is often misused and misunderstood. Nonetheless, for ease of language I will use both terms.

A problematic substance for your individual body might be something you ingest, inhale or absorb. There are substances that are problematic for all people, such as DDT (a pesticide) was shown to be, while there are others that are specific to an individual. For example, gluten behaves as a problematic substance for some people.

Their road into the body might vary, but once they are in the blood, the body has to deal with them, as problematic substances cannot be allowed to accumulate in the blood. So the body shunts them to the liver and the kidneys for detoxification (transformation into something less harmful that can be excreted), filtration and then excretion. For the liver and kidneys to perform their critical work, nutrients are required.

But here's the thing: if the load arriving at the front door of either of these organs is too much for it to deal with at the time, due to the previous ongoing loads being too much or too regular, the problematic substances still need to be removed from the blood so that they don't harm you. In such cases they are moved to the fatty tissues of our body (unfortunately some are stored in bone or brain as well), away from the vital organs, and the fat cells become storage houses for toxins.

Your body is geared for survival. To burn the stored fat as fuel and hence lose weight, you will also need to release these stored toxins, and your body can only do that when it has the required detoxification and filtration capacity. This means you need to put fewer problematic substances in, and enhance your nutritional status through increasing the nutrient density of your diet. Not eat fewer calories! Moreover, if the low-calorie foods come out of packets, they potentially contain some problematic substances.

If you don't create the space for your liver to have to do less detoxification work by decreasing the loaders going in, and you don't increase the nutrients you ingest to allow the liver to create more enzymes required for the critical detoxification work, then fat won't be burnt as you are not freeing up the required detoxification capacity.

It is not a pleasant thing to consider, nor for the people who experience this, but essentially people are getting more and more toxic due to their lifestyle choices, and due to a lack of awareness about the chemical load going into their bodies via what they eat, drink, inhale from the air, or absorb through the skin.

The calorie equation doesn't have a toxicity factor, and science currently has no way of calculating this. The fact remains that, even if you eat fewer calories than you burn, but the calories going in are not from whole, real, nutrient-dense foods, your body will still not have the resources to allow you to burn your body fat and enable you to lose weight. For to do so, risks dumping the problematic substances back into your blood, which could harm you in a minor or major way. And your body is so clever it won't allow this to happen so instead it will continue to store the toxins until it can process them. Meanwhile, you will keep getting frustrated that you are making all of this effort and your clothes still won't be getting any looser.

The Gallbladder

Another key factor to the body being able to detoxify and eliminate potentially problematic substances is the efficiency of the gallbladder to release bile. The liver produces bile. Many toxins are fat-soluble, and bile is essential for them to be metabolized, detoxified and eliminated.

Good bile production and release occurs as part of the cascade of signals that is generated from good digestion. If stomach acid production is poor or if the pH is too high (not acidic enough to initiate the pH gradient of the digestive tract), for the variety of reasons discussed in the "Foundation of Nourishment" section, bile release from the gallbladder can be compromised. Gall stones can be another reason for the gallbladder not working optimally. Bitter foods and herbs stimulate bile production, which is not a flavour many people seek out.

For those who have had their gallbladder removed, the liver has to continue to make the bile the gallbladder is no longer available to store, asking the liver to jump to action more frequently and accomplish yet another task on its long list. Producing bile is not the liver's only job, plus it cannot make as much bile without the gallbladder as the body has nowhere to store the bile. This means that those who have had their gallbladder removed need to take extra good care of their liver for the liver to be highly responsive to the need for bile so that poor-quality fats and fat-based toxins are able to be detoxified and eliminated efficiently from the body.

If someone has a fatty liver (explained in the "Detox Engine" and "Fat Storage, Sugar and Appetite" sections), they can follow a plan of action designed for them by a health professional experienced in this area, to allow the liver to start to release some of the stored fat.

It will come away in bowel motions as a fatty film, or globules of oil may be visible after a motion. I know it's no fun to talk about this, but I want this information to be clear.

> focus on the body systems that need support, based on the symptoms an individual is presenting with.

All of the above is partly why whenever someone seeks me out for assistance with weight loss, I don't focus on the weight. I have never weighed a client, something I explain in *Accidentally Overweight*. I focus on the body systems that need support, based on the symptoms an individual is presenting with. This is also why with any weight loss programme anyone ever undertakes in this world we now live in, it needs to be accompanied by liver support, either through the diet, green drinks, nutrient supplementation and/or herbal medicine.

◈ Fat Cells and Toxicity In Short ... _____

Adipose tissue:

- ◆ is another name for body fat
- ◆ is not just fatty tissue, it also functions like a gland
- ◆ makes oestrogen in both men and women
- ◆ stores toxins
- ◆ will not be used as fuel (ie, calories burnt) if the body does not have the capacity to detoxify the toxins that may be released when the fat gets utilized
- ◆ sometimes requires the person to undertake diet and lifestyle changes that support the liver so that body fat can be readily utilized efficiently as a fuel.

Why Eat Organic?

One way I want to encourage people to eat is to not only move away from refined and processed foods, but also to decrease the synthetic chemical load through encouraging the consumption of more organically or biodynamically grown food. Choosing more spray-free options is also viable in achieving this.

It is my opinion that we are guinea pigs when it comes to the long-term consumption of pesticides. The reason a conventionally grown apple looks so perfect is because it has been sprayed to make it that way. We cannot see or taste the chemicals on its skin, but they are there. Pesticides have to be tested before they can be used on food for human consumption. However, they are often tested for such a relatively brief amount of time that I do not believe we can compare tests done over, say, a six-month period, to being exposed to these substances over an entire lifetime. What also cannot be tested is what happens when the chemicals are mixed, and they get mixed inside our body every day when we eat conventionally grown produce.

Fresh food the way it comes in Nature is an incredibly important part of our diet. Please do not be scared off from eating a conventionally farmed apple. I simply want to encourage you to choose organic produce whenever you can. Also, think about the way you eat the food. We peel a banana. It may have been sprayed, but how much gets through the skin? We actually don't know. But surely there would be less chemical residue in the flesh of a banana than on the skin. So perhaps choosing a conventionally grown banana is not too bad. No one really knows. Yet, when it comes to an apple, we usually eat the whole fruit. So you would be better to choose an organic (or biodynamically grown) apple wherever possible.

Think about this: organic food is the true cost of food. I once started and ran an organic café. Once a week, a local farmer delivered fresh greens picked that morning from his biodynamic farm. I always set aside some time on the day of his delivery to chat with him, as he always had wonderful tales to tell of life on his farm. One day, when I asked him how he was, his reply was along the lines of "not so good". When I enquired further, he told me that snails had invaded his broccoli patch, virtually overnight. When I paused to consider this, I realized that, if they took hold, a portion of this man's meagre livelihood would be lost. So I asked him how he deals with snails on his broccoli, given that his farming principles do not involve spraying the patch to get rid of the invaders (which would have taken less than 30 minutes to do).

My farmer friend went on to tell me that snails lose their "stick", their ability to suction onto things, in salty water. So he made up a bottle of salt and water, and he spent two days, crouched down on all fours, crawling between his broccoli plants, squirting saline water up under the fronds. Not only that, he didn't kill the snails, he collected them in a bucket and fed them to the chooks "to keep them in the food chain", as he so delightfully put it.

Think about each of these scenarios. Spray in under 30 minutes versus crawling around on your haunches for two days. For me, that illustrates precisely why organic and biodynamic food costs more. It reflects the real cost of food; plus many foods grown this way have a greater nutritional value simply from how the soil has been tended. If a nutrient is not in the soil, it cannot be in the food. The more of us who choose organic or biodynamic food, the cheaper it will become. Every time you spend money, you are casting a vote for the kind of world you want. The more we demand organic and say no to synthetic chemicals, the more organics will have to be supplied. So choose organic food whenever you can.

If organic food is simply not available in your area or it is too costly for you to buy, try this solution to remove pesticides.

Pesticides tend to be fat-soluble, so general washing does not remove them. Washing food can remove dirt and germs, but not most pesticides. To wash food for both dirt and pesticides at the same time, fill your sink with three parts water to one part vinegar, and wash your fruits and vegetables. Then rinse them in fresh water, pat them dry, and store them for use. Do what is practical for you.

Furthermore, plants have innate mechanisms designed to help them protect themselves from pests. When a plant is left to grow of its accord and is not sprayed with pesticides, the plant creates substances within itself to help ward off pests. However, these substances don't just have the ability to help protect the plant, they often behave as antioxidants when humans consume them. If the plants are sprayed, they no longer have to (and don't) produce these substances that enhance human health. So eating organic food is not just about what you miss out on (pesticides), but also what you get (more antioxidants).

Pesticides, being fat-soluble, typically have to be altered inside the body before they can be excreted. The liver is one

> *E*ating organic food is not just about what you miss out on (pesticides), but also what you get (more antioxidants).

organ involved in this process. The liver has to prioritize detoxification processes, and so if there are more liver-loaders present than available pathways for this to occur, the pesticides are usually stored in the fatty tissue of your body. Hence when any weight-loss process is undertaken, liver support is of immense importance, as these substances become mobilized.

On another note, some herbicides contain compounds that can mimic oestrogen in the human body, in both males and females of all ages. This is of great concern. For oestrogen or oestrogen-like compounds to exert their effects, they have to bind to oestrogen receptors, and when they do, the lovely or not-so-lovely effects of oestrogen are felt. Given that children today are exposed to herbicides for their entire lifetimes, it is likely that their exposure to oestrogen-like compounds in addition to what the body makes itself, mostly from puberty onwards, is contributing to the earlier age of menarche being reported across the Western world. Pause and consider the ramifications of this.

Decrease your regular intake of synthetic chemicals by choosing organic produce or growing some of your own food, such as herbs, wherever you can. However, if this overwhelms you, don't start your lifestyle changes here. Come to this when you are ready. In the meantime, focus on enhancing your nutritional intake through eating more real food and consuming fewer substances that have the potential to take away from your health, such as those found in processed foods.

It is very difficult to be patient and kind with yourself and others, when you are filling yourself with stimulants such as too much caffeine, and eating a diet high in processed foods that is virtually devoid of nutrients.

Dr Libby

Detox Engine

The health and efficiency of the liver plays a significant role in whether we lose body fat or not, yet it is another factor not considered in any of the energy equations. I believe that the decisions the liver makes are some of the most critical to our health and longevity, and whether we burn fat or store it.

When it comes to every aspect of our health, the liver packs a mighty punch. It is one of the big guns when it comes to your energy, vitality and hormonal balance, as well as to the clarity of your skin and eyes. In conjunction with the gallbladder, the liver works endlessly to help us excrete fatty substances that the body no longer needs, including old hormones, pesticides and stored body fat.

The liver is the body's second largest organ after our skin. It sits behind your right ribcage. Its primary role is detoxification, a concept that has had much confusion surrounding it — confusion I want to resolve for you.

How the Liver Works and Signs of Poor Functioning

A simple way to imagine the detoxification power of the liver is to picture a triangle shape: inside that triangle are billions and billions of little circles, each one of them a liver cell. Imagine that inside each liver cell is a mouse on a wheel, running and running and running, with each turn of the billions of little wheels driving your liver function. When we treat our liver unkindly, a circle can die, and for a time the liver can regenerate a new cell to replace the dead cell, but after a while this is no longer possible, and a globule of fat can take up residence where once that fat-burning little "mouse" was working.

When many fat globules take over (known as "fatty liver"), our health can suffer significantly. Less efficient detoxification processes can lead to poor thyroid function, sex hormone imbalances, congested skin, lousy cholesterol, and impaired blood glucose management that often shows up as sugar cravings. Moreover, where our body wants to lay down body fat can also shift. For the first time people may notice that they have a fat roll quite high up on their abdomen. For women this is just below their bra line, and for men, just beneath their pectoral muscles. It can come and go, and sometimes there is a point right in the centre of the torso that is tender. I will always suggest ways to support your liver based on the presence of a fat roll in that position, and gallbladder support based on that tender point. Sometimes both organs need support. In the not-too-distant past, only people who regularly over-consumed alcohol developed fatty liver disease, but now we are seeing teenagers develop it simply from eating diets high in processed foods. This has become so common, that a new disease has been named, called "non-alcoholic fatty liver disease". Imagine a liver that looks just like one that has been chronically battered by alcohol, but processed food has created it.

Detoxification

It is important you understand the mechanisms of detoxification and elimination that your body utilizes, because, when they are compromised, whether we burn body fat or store it can also be influenced. There are numerous organs and body systems involved in detoxification. They include:

- the *liver* transforms substances that if they were to accumulate would harm you, altering them into less harmful substances you can then excrete
- the *colon* (digestive system) contains bacteria that produce both healthy and unhealthy substances, so you want to keep your bowel moving regularly, as one of its roles is to release waste and problematic substances so they don't accumulate

> *D*etoxification is essentially a transformation process. Any substance that would be harmful to you if it accumulated in your body must be changed into a less harmful form so that it can then be excreted safely from your body.

* the *kidneys* are constantly filtering your blood and getting rid of anything you don't need, including toxins, in urine

* the *skin* not only protects and houses your organs, but it allows problematic substances to leave the body via perspiration

* the *respiratory system* plays a key role in the detoxification squad — even the hairs inside your nose help filter the air you breathe in — while the lungs are responsible for filtering out fumes, allergens, mould, and airborne toxins; when we are stressed, we tend to shift from slow belly-breathing to short, shallow upper-chest breaths, which in turn can reduce the lungs' ability to transport oxygen to all tissues; for those of you who know my work, you now know another reason (other than the nervous system and stress-hormone-lowering benefits) why diaphragmatic breathing is my number one health tip.

Detoxification is a process that goes on inside us all day, every day. The choices we make influence how efficiently the liver is able to do its job. Detoxification is essentially a transformation process. Any substance that would be harmful to you if it accumulated in your body must be changed into a less harmful form so that it can then be excreted safely from your body. To look and feel your best, you want this to be a highly efficient process.

There are two stages to the detoxification process, appropriately named phase 1 and phase 2 liver detoxification. Both phases require certain nutrients to function, and dietary choices can influence how efficiently each phase is able to work. The figure below illustrates the phases of detoxification, and you can see some of the nutrients that are required.

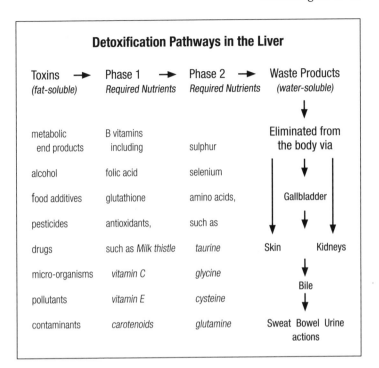

Liver detoxification pathways: Phase 1 and phase 2 liver detoxification pathways, and the nutrients essential to these vital processes.

Phase 1

For the first stage of detoxification, numerous nutrients, including B vitamins, are essential. Whole grains are one of the richest sources of B vitamins we have in the food supply; however, many people feel much better with fewer or none of these foods in their diets. People decrease or cut grains out of their diets for varied reasons. Some first experienced rapid weight loss with the advent of the high-protein, very low-carbohydrate diets, purported as the ultimate answer to weight-loss desires in the late 1990s, a repeat of the popular dietary concept from the 1970s, and a natural progression from the high-carbohydrate, low-fat guidelines that had preceded them. Others simply started to notice that foods made from grains induced reflux or made their tummy bloated, and they took action to change how they felt. If grains feel good for you and energize you, then enjoy them in whole food form; some are best soaked prior to consumption. If they don't suit you, don't eat them. Your body knows best what works for you. Simply be aware that if you have a low intake of B vitamins, your phase 1 liver detoxification processes may not function optimally. It can be useful to take a supplement if you eat a low-carbohydrate diet or avoid/limit grains.

Phase 2

There is one road into the liver and five pathways out of the liver. Just as for phase 1 reactions, phase 2 liver pathways also require certain nutrients to function, in particular, specific amino acids and sulphur.

We get our amino acids from protein foods. Think about this next statement: what we eat becomes part of us. Protein foods are broken down into amino acids, and they go on to create all of the cells of your immune system, which are what defends you from infection. Amino acids also go on to create the neurotransmitters in your brain that influence your mood and your clarity of thought. They also build your pretty muscles that allow you to carry your groceries. What you eat really does matter — your food becomes part of you.

For further phase 2 support we need sulphur which we obtain from eggs, onion, garlic and shallots, as well as from the *Brassica* family of vegetables, which includes broccoli, cabbage, kale, Brussels sprouts, and cauliflower. The liver makes enzymes that are responsible for the transformation of each substance, and the rate of production of these essential enzymes determines how quickly each substance is processed. The load placed on the liver also determines how quickly things move through the liver, and you will see shortly how all of this impacts on how you look and feel, as well as how your clothes fit you. I believe it is one of the biggest reasons why the calorie equation is redundant in today's world.

Liver-loaders

There is a group of substances I lovingly label "liver-loaders". They include:

- alcohol
- caffeine
- trans fats
- refined sugars
- synthetic substances, such as pesticides, medications, skincare products
- infection; for example, viruses such as glandular fever (also known as Epstein–Barr virus, mononucleosis).

When we consider our exposure to synthetic substances we must consider skincare. We are crazy if we think that we don't absorb things through our skin. You only have to look at the way nicotine patches work to realize that the skin provides a direct route to our blood stream, carrying the blood that the liver will need to "clean". There are plenty of wonderful skincare companies out there who do not use synthetic ingredients. Seek them out or even make your own. I love to suggest to people that it would be good if they could eat their skincare! You want to be able to recognize the words on the label of your skincare, just as you do with food.

It is also important to do what we can to minimize our exposure to, and consumption of, pesticides and herbicides. Firstly, a number of these synthetic chemicals mimic oestrogen and can bind to the oestrogen receptors in the body, which has consequences for males and females of all ages. Research from the United States suggests that for 40% of girls in the United States, the average age of onset of menstruation is now eight years. It is difficult to explain how this is so without contemplating the role of environmental oestrogens.

As discussed in the "Why Eat Organic?" section, another concern with the consumption of pesticides and herbicides is the risk of their storage in the fatty tissue of our body. We don't know the long-term consequences of this, or of being exposed to these substances for an entire lifetime, as we are essentially the first generation of people to be exposed to some of them for such a long period. Do we yet know the extent of their cumulative impact on metabolism, let alone other aspects of our health?

Internal Stressors

However, it is not just infections or the things we consume or put on our skin that can place demands on the detoxification processes of the liver. Substances your body makes itself also need transformation by the liver so that they can be excreted. These substances include:

cholesterol

steroid (sex) hormones, such as oestrogen

substances created by or causing any short-fall in digestion, due to compromised digestive processes, as explored in the "Foundation of Nourishment" section

untreated food sensitivities

undiagnosed coeliac disease.

I have met countless people who have not consumed much in the way of liver-loaders, but have diabolical menstrual cycles or an ongoing challenge with irritable bowel syndrome or constipation, and who often exhibit what I consider to be distinct signs that their liver needs support. Passing clots while menstruating is a classic liver congestion sign, as are many skin conditions. More symptoms are listed below.

Indications Your Liver Needs Support

The following are symptoms that may indicate that your liver needs support:

liver roll

a tender point in the centre of your torso (which can indicate gallbladder issues, past emotional heartbreak, or massive

disappointment); if your gallbladder has been removed, your liver has to make the bile on demand as the gallbladder is no longer there to store it, so additional liver support is often required

* short fuse or bad temper
* episodes or feelings of intense anger
* "liverish", gritty, impatient behaviour
* premenstrual syndrome
* cellulite (lymphatic or cortisol-related also)
* congested skin or skin outbreaks related to the menstrual cycle
* skin rashes
* eczema, rosacea
* overheating easily
* "floaters" in your vision (can also be a sign of iron deficiency)
* waking around 2am
* poor sleep on an evening you consume alcohol
* waking up hot during the night
* not hungry for breakfast when you first get up in the morning
* preference for coffee to start your day
* elevated cholesterol
* oestrogen-dominance symptoms
* bloating easily
* daily alcohol consumption
* daily long-term caffeine consumption (although tea and green tea are more favourable than coffee, soft drinks and energy drinks).

Cholesterol

Cholesterol is an extremely important substance. We only ever hear bad press about cholesterol; however, we would melt without it. It is the building block of all of our steroid hormones, including progesterone and testosterone. The process that cholesterol undergoes to form steroid hormones is illustrated in the diagram below.

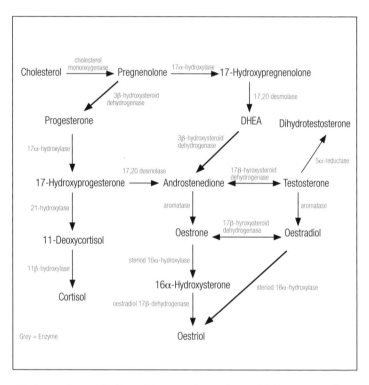

Cholesterol metabolism: The creation of steroid hormones from cholesterol.

The reason I include the above biochemical diagram is to illustrate the way substances in the body flow onward to create other substances. Only some of the cholesterol that the body makes, or that you obtain from your diet, remains as cholesterol, and much of that is required for healthy brain function. Twenty-five per cent of the body's cholesterol is stored in the brain and plays a critical role there. You do not want too much cholesterol accumulating as cholesterol in your blood, although I anticipate conventional medicine will soon increase what they consider to be "safe" blood cholesterol levels. You want your cholesterol metabolism to be efficient and able to regulate itself, which it can with healthy liver function. You want some of the cholesterol to turn into progesterone, testosterone, DHEA and oestrogen. All of the words in the diagram that begin with "Oest" are different forms of oestrogen.

Your diet contributes to approximately 20% of the amount of cholesterol in your blood, while your liver creates the other 80%. Your liver tends to make extra cholesterol when it needs to protect itself, as cholesterol behaves like an anti-inflammatory in certain situations. What are some of the things that may inflame the liver and drive additional cholesterol production? The liver-loaders listed above. One of the most successful ways to manage your blood level of cholesterol is to take extra good care of your liver and deal with any inflammation in the body. The source or sources of the inflammation ideally need to be identified and removed, if possible, and adding some anti-inflammatory essential fats can be invaluable. You may decide to start with a good-quality essential fatty acid supplement.

To illustrate the immense power of your liver: there is not one person in 16 years whose cholesterol I haven't lowered back into the normal range simply by guiding them to take care of their liver. Over time, I have also witnessed the other incredible health benefits that unfold when we focus on taking care of our liver, and weight loss — not due to fewer calories and more exercise — is the most common. For me, elevated cholesterol is simply one way the body communicates that the liver needs some additional support.

Healthy Cholesterol Metabolism

Healthy cholesterol metabolism is best imagined as a gently flowing stream. You want a small amount of cholesterol to remain in your blood as cholesterol, but you want the rest to do its critical work in the brain and also to be converted into your sex (steroid) hormones. Men and women make all three of the major sex hormones: testosterone, oestrogen and progesterone. Each gender makes them in differing ratios, with men producing more testosterone and far less oestrogen, along with some progesterone, while women make more oestrogen and progesterone and less testosterone. You can see from the diagram that certain enzymes push the hormones one way or the other.

Cholesterol levels

Sometimes over time, however, too much cholesterol can accumulate as cholesterol. To come back to the analogy of cholesterol metabolism being like a flowing stream, it is as though a dam wall gets built across the flow and, instead of cholesterol being converted into sex hormones, it accumulates in the blood as cholesterol. There are two problems here.

One is that too much blood cholesterol may pose a health problem. Although the jury is still out on whether this is actually true from a heart disease perspective, my opinion is that cholesterol is not related to heart disease, and science is starting to show that the original conclusions drawn from the research linking cholesterol and heart disease were most likely incorrect. Cholesterol is only a problem in your blood if the wall of a blood vessel is damaged by a free radical, which occurs if there aren't enough antioxidants present to pair up with the free radical, or if there is elevated blood glucose or homocysteine, as this leads cholesterol to become sticky and act like a plaster covering and protecting the site of the damage.

The other is that you now have lower levels of sex hormones being produced. Your steroid hormones make you feel vital and alive. They are an enormous contributing factor to whether you bounce or stagger out of bed each morning, and whether your skin is free from blemishes, and glows. When your sex hormones are balanced and at optimal levels, you feel amazing.

Dietary factors

For cholesterol to be converted into sex hormones, you must have optimal zinc levels, and essential fatty acids are also important. Our best sources of the omega-3 fats are the oils in fish, flaxseeds (linseeds), walnuts and pecans, while evening primrose oil and borage oil are good sources of the essential fats of the omega-6 type. The richest food source of zinc is oysters. Beef and lamb also contain zinc, and our vegetable sources include seeds, such as sunflower seeds and pumpkin seeds.

As far as amounts go, oysters contain 70 milligrams of zinc per 100 grams, while beef, being the next best source of zinc, contains only 4 milligrams per 100 grams. Lamb has on average 2.9 milligrams of zinc per 100 grams, while seeds have around 0.9 milligrams of zinc per 100 grams. In the not-so-distant past, we obtained consistent amounts of zinc from our plant foods. But food is only as good as the quality of the soil in which it is grown, and if a nutrient is not in the soil then it cannot be in our food. Most soil in the Western world is deficient in zinc unless it has been organically or — better still, from a zinc perspective — biodynamically farmed.

Each adult needs a minimum of 15 milligrams of zinc per day just so the body can perform its basic functions. That is potentially not even enough for optimal health. So from where on Earth are we getting our zinc? The answer is that many of us are not. Some studies have suggested that up to 70% of people living in Western countries are potentially deficient in zinc, and it is a mineral that is not only essential for keeping cholesterol levels in check and producing optimal amounts of sex hormones, but is also vital to skin health and wound healing, as well as digestion and immune function. Zinc is a mighty little mineral.

Cholesterol excretion
The second part of this biochemical picture about cholesterol metabolism and liver health involves the excretion of cholesterol. The same mechanism also applies to oestrogen, an issue to consider for both men and women. It is of particular importance for any females who read the section about sex hormones and identify oestrogen dominance.

When a liver-loader, either consumed (*exogenous*) or made as a result of internal chemistry (*endogenous*), arrives at the front door of the liver, it has arrived to be transformed. (In the explanation that follows, let's remain focused on cholesterol as the liver-loader, so the mechanism is clear.) So when any of the liver-loaders arrive at the front door of the liver, they undergo their first stage of change (phase 1 liver detoxification). Between the front door and the middle of the liver, cholesterol is still cholesterol, but it has been altered somewhat. This slightly changed cholesterol then wants to go down one of the five phase 2 detox roads, and, once it has done that, it has been slightly altered again, and it is this substance that can then be excreted — expelled from your body forever.

Health problems can arise, however, when the traffic on the phase 2 pathways gets banked up like traffic on a motorway. After years of regularly consumed liver-loaders, and/or hormonal or bowel problems, the roads out of the liver can become congested. Conventional blood tests for liver function do not reveal this. The liver usually takes years of battering before conventional blood tests reflect the congestion that led to them becoming elevated in the first place. When the traffic is banked up, the cholesterol (or oestrogen), undergoes its first stage of change and arrives in the middle of the liver, ready to go down its appropriate path for the second stage of transformation it must undergo before it can be excreted. If the phase 2 pathways are congested, the cholesterol (or oestrogen) sitting in the middle of the liver has nowhere to go, but it cannot remain waiting in the middle of the liver, as there is more rubbish constantly coming through the front door of the liver. When this occurs, the liver releases the cholesterol, or oestrogen, back out into the blood, where it gets recycled. It is the recycling of these substances, not the substances themselves, that can potentially be harmful to human health, including our waistlines due to the metabolic effects that increased levels of these substances generate. What organ can we take much better care of if we want to stop this recycling from happening? Our precious liver. Our livers need more support, and less of a load, for amazing energy, vitality and weight loss.

On another note, and as you will see in the "Hormone Havoc" section, it is the recycled form of oestrogen that is of such concern for women regarding the risk of developing reproductive cancers. Oestrogen is a beautiful hormone in the right amount and with the right types of oestrogen in a balanced ratio. Too much total oestrogen or too much of the type linked to reproductive cancers are the problems; not only because of the oestrogen itself, but also because progesterone production can never match it. That latter scenario alone can impact whether you burn fat or store it.

Antioxidant Defence Mechanisms

Another way the body detoxifies, other than through phase 1 and 2 detoxification pathways, is through our antioxidant defence mechanisms. This is a superb aspect of our chemistry. Humans stay alive through a process called *respiration*, meaning that we breathe in oxygen, and we exhale carbon dioxide. If you could see oxygen in space, it is two Os (oxygen molecules) stuck together. The diagram below illustrates what I will describe.

$$O_2$$
$$O = O$$
$$O^- \text{ (free radical)}$$
$$A/O \text{ (antioxidant/donator)}$$
$$O = O$$
$$O_2$$

Free radical protection from antioxidants: The oxygen donation of antioxidants.

When we breathe, oxygen splits apart, forming two single oxygen molecules. Known as *free radicals*, they have the potential to damage your tissues. One of the major ways the body defends itself from damage by a free radical is through the consumption of antioxidants. Antioxidant-rich foods are our coloured plant foods. Blueberries, green tea, red wine and chocolate (cacao) are rich in antioxidants, and are the most common antioxidant-rich foods called out at my live events when I ask the audience for ideas. As the skins and seeds of the red grapes are especially high in antioxidants, grape juice is just as powerful as red wine (from an antioxidant perspective), and doesn't ask the liver to do extra detox work. The antioxidant donates one of its oxygens back to the free radical, and they pair up. Oxygen is then content again, and damage to your tissues is avoided. We generate more free radicals in response to our exposure to pollution and anything that increases respiration.

To understand one powerful way free radicals can damage our tissues, imagine a blood vessel leading to your heart. A free radical zips about through the blood and suddenly does a dive-bomb and makes an indentation in the wall of the vessel. It resembles the divot in the grass beneath a golf swing that has taken too much soil with it. The damaged vessel sends out a cry for help, signalling that it is damaged, and, in this case, cholesterol wants to be the hero. Cholesterol behaves like a band-aid in this situation, and it comes along and sticks itself on top of the injured site. It then sends out a message to all of its cholesterol friends to join the band-aid party, and they come along and stick themselves over the top of the first cholesterol globule that arrived. The cholesterol piles up, and it oxidizes and hardens. This is called atherosclerosis or plaque, and it narrows the interior of the arteries. Where once the blood could flow through a wide, open vessel, it now has a very narrow, restricted path to weave. Your blood is the only way oxygen and nutrients get around your body. Your heart is a muscle, and it needs both oxygen and nutrients to survive. If it is starved of either of these for long enough, this is one mechanism that can lead to a heart attack.

The good news, though, is that this condition is reversible. The hardened, built-up cholesterol is *LDL cholesterol*, which is why it is commonly known as "bad" cholesterol. "Good" cholesterol (*HDL cholesterol*) comes along and unsticks each globule of cholesterol and carries it off to — guess where? You guessed it: the liver. It arrives at the front door of the liver to undergo its detoxification process and, when the liver is functioning well, the cholesterol is processed, excreted and gone forever. However, as outlined previously, if the liver is loaded up with substances that it *must* prioritize higher up the detox order than boring old, homemade cholesterol, then the cholesterol reaches the midpoint of the liver, is released too soon, and gets reabsorbed. This is one way our blood cholesterol goes up and up and up. Cholesterol can also be elevated when thyroid function is poor.

Alcohol

I cannot conclude talking about liver detoxification without talking about liver-loader number one: alcohol. There is a reason it is at the top of the list — I consider it one of the most pervasive substances impacting too many livers today. I see people who might eat as green as can be, but at the same time consume alcohol daily. Alcohol is certainly a substance that can take away our vitality, and sometimes the vitality of those around us, particularly when it is regularly over-consumed. As a society, we need to get real about the dangers of routine alcohol consumption. Weight that won't shift can be a major consequence, too, particularly if the regular over-consumption has been going on longer-term, and this is not necessarily due to alcohol's calorie content. Because of the way alcohol is broken down in the body, requiring the liver to transform the alcohol into acetaldehyde before it can be excreted, it can lead to sex hormone imbalances due to oestrogen recycling; hello, fat storage. Many alcoholic drinks are also very high in sugars (carbohydrates) and hence require insulin; hi again, fat storage. It also leads to excess cortisol production and — you guessed it — another fat-storage signalling message to the body. You can see how far more than the calorie equation is at work in this scenario.

The effects of the regular over-consumption of alcohol are wide-reaching. Whether it is increased body fat or cellulite, less energy, worse bouts of PMS, or mood fluctuations ... or perhaps your get-up-and-go has got up and left, the price of over-consumption is just not worth it. As fun as it can be at the time, alcohol can rob you of your clarity and purpose when it is regularly over-consumed.

January often sees people making big statements about their health, and alcohol reduction or avoidance. Some wait until February to take a break, as they have worked out that it has the least number of days! I know others who do Dry July or Oct-sober. Others simply select the special occasions when they choose to imbibe, rather than making it part of every day or totally going without.

We drink for wide and varied reasons. For some, it is the way they socialize, or the way they wind down from the day. Some use alcohol to distract themselves from thoughts and feelings they would rather avoid, and to numb themselves from registering that there are things about their life they would like to change. It can be a way for people to cope. Regardless of the reason, too many people overdrink without even realizing it.

A standard drink is 100 grams of alcohol, in whatever form that comes. In Australia and New Zealand, 100 grams of alcohol is a 330-millilitre bottle of 4% beer, a 30-millilitre nip of spirits, 170 millilitres of champagne, or a measly 100 millilitres of wine — about four swallows! Next time you pour yourself a glass of wine, measure it, and see what your natural pour is. For most, it is considerably more than 100 millilitres, and, as a result, many people unknowingly over-drink.

The current recommendations provided by the Australian Heart Foundation in concurrence with the National Health and Medical Research Council (NHMRC) now suggest for those who already drink alcohol it is safe to consume no more than two standard drinks per day for both men and women. Other organizations add that the evidence suggests that that must include two alcohol-free days (AFDs) per week. However, I also encourage you to consider the position statement on alcohol endorsed by many of the cancer organizations from around the world, which says that if you have a family history of cancer, there is no safe level of alcohol consumption — which is a very powerful statement to contemplate.

I am not suggesting that you don't drink. Having a drink can be immensely pleasurable for those who partake on occasions. I simply want to appeal to you to get honest with yourself about how alcohol may affect you. You know in your heart if you drink too much and when it is negatively impacting your health. Alcohol can affect the way we relate to those we love the most in the world, and of course it affects how we feel about ourselves. So, if you drink, drink for the pleasure of it or to celebrate on occasions, rather than to escape from your daily life.

The link between the consistent over-consumption of alcohol and breast cancer is undeniable. Research has shown this time and time again and for many years now. Yet, we rarely hear about it.

As we have learnt, the human body cannot excrete alcohol; it has to be converted into acetaldehyde by the liver, and then the acetaldehyde can be excreted. This is the nasty substance that can accumulate, and is what gives us a headache or hangover after excessive consumption. If the liver doesn't do its job properly and alcohol accumulates in our blood, we can fall into a coma and die. Alcohol is a poison to the human body, but, thankfully, our liver usually jumps to action and starts the conversion process and we can carry on. Over time, though, this takes its toll.

When we drink daily, or, for some, just regularly, the liver can be so busy dealing with alcohol as its priority that other substances the liver has to change so they can be excreted don't get any attention and are recycled. Oestrogen and cholesterol are two examples. It is often the reabsorption of these substances that leads to elevated levels in our body, and that can lead to more significant health challenges and weight that is difficult to shift.

If you want to cut back or cut out alcohol for a while, or even if you just want to break your habit of regular drinking, still pour yourself a drink at the time you would normally have a glass of wine, and do what you would normally do. Sit and chat to your partner, make dinner, talk on the phone to a friend. So often we have mentally linked the glass of wine to a pleasurable activity when it is actually the pleasurable activity that we don't want to miss out on! So have sparkling water in a wine glass, with some fresh lime or lemon if that appeals, and add a few more AFDs to your life.

Liver Support

At the weekend events that I run, I help people understand the guilt that a vicious cycle of too much alcohol in the evenings, coffee to cope the next morning and sugar cravings mid-afternoon drives. The guilt you feel tends to lead you back to that cycle whereas if you saw it as a one-off and then returned to a higher level of self-care, it would have a much more minimal impact. Remember, it is what you do every day that impacts on your health, not what you do sometimes.

Be honest with yourself about the liver-loaders in your life. Focus on taking good care of yourself and nourishing yourself, rather than on what you may need to consume less of. As you have read, the liver plays a significant role in the metabolism of countless substances that are linked to whether the body gets the message to burn body fat or store it, processes not factored into the calorie equation. If you eat well and move regularly and nothing ever changes with your body shape or size, you may find it highly beneficial to start focusing on liver support. We only have one liver. Love it accordingly.

✦ Detox Engine In Short ... _____

Your liver has many roles, one of which is detoxification, a transformation process that occurs essentially in two stages: namely, phase 1 and phase 2. Both stages require a specific range of nutrients, and if any of these are deficient, detoxification will not be efficient and may be impaired. Poor liver detoxification processes can lead to weight gain, hence a nutrient-dense diet is critical for optimal liver function.

If there are too many "liver-loaders" requiring detoxification, the traffic moving through the liver can become banked up like traffic on a motorway. This can lead to problematic substances, such as slightly changed forms of oestrogen, being recycled. This slightly changed form of oestrogen has been highly linked to women's reproductive system cancers and breast cancer. Oestrogen is also linked to fat storage signals for the body, and oestrogen dominance has, for some, been found to inhibit fat burning and hence weight loss. Therefore, part of the link between poor liver detoxification and an inability to lose weight is due to the metabolic consequences of the problematic substances (toxins) the liver recycles.

Another way the liver can impair fat loss that is not down to the calorie equation is through what is known as a fatty liver. If the detoxification pathways become overloaded, the toxic substances can start to build up in the blood, but, as this is too dangerous to your survival, they are moved to and accumulate in the fatty tissues and organs. This can result in symptoms of hormonal imbalances, such as breast pain, menstrual cycle dysregulation and/or pain, pre-menstrual syndrome (PMS), early or debilitating menopause, and reduced sperm count in men, as well as weight that won't budge.

If the liver detoxification pathways become overloaded, toxins, fat globules, dead cells and microorganisms can build up in the blood to undesirably high levels. This asks the immune system to do more work, and it can become overloaded. This leads the immune system to produce excessive inflammatory substances, and in some cases auto-antibodies due to it constantly being stimulated. This can lead to symptoms of immune dysfunction, all too common today, such as allergies, inflammatory diseases, recurrent infections, and autoimmune diseases. Other processes can lead to these immune system conditions, but ongoing long-term poor liver detoxification is often one of the major contributing factors.

Liver cells have an incredible ability to replace themselves when they are damaged, but when the damage just keeps on coming they are eventually no longer able to do this, and a globule of fat will replace where a functioning liver cell once was. Once fat starts to take up residence in the liver, detoxification is compromised and people gain weight, whether their calorie equation has changed or not.

A fatty liver that was once only seen in chronic alcoholics is now being found in scans of teenagers who have never consumed alcohol, simply as a result of the amount of processed foods and drinks they consume. The liver just can't keep up with what too many people ask of it today. Thousands of people over my working life will tell me they "only have two glasses of wine" each night. Two glasses for many people is half a bottle, as they share it with their partner. With wine, you get four liver-loaders: alcohol, preservatives, pesticides (as grapes are one of the most highly sprayed crops) and refined sugar, half of which is fructose, as well as the sugars from the grapes. If these things were all spread out on a plate for you to eat, I doubt you would swallow them with so much enthusiasm, and you certainly would not do this nightly. If you swallow what wine is made of every night for 5 or 20 or 50 years, your liver will let you know of its discomfort in some way. Perhaps find an organic wine with no preservatives and remove two of the liver-loaders as a starting point and/or add some more AFDs to your week.

A fatty liver can be reversed, and with it comes weight loss, if there is weight to lose. I have seen this occur in thousands of clients over the years, with not one calorie counted, and not one piece of food weighed. When you supply your body with foods that nourish it — with real, whole foods and drinks — you do two things. First, you supply the body with the nutrients it needs for outstanding liver detoxification, and secondly, you are omitting the non-food ingredients that can be present in many processed foods that add to the liver's workload. I will say it again: if you need to count anything, count nutrients.

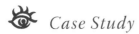 *Case Study*

Sarah's Story

Sarah was 23 when she came to see me about her skin. She was very self-conscious about her pimples, but didn't want to go on medication to treat them. I explained that the skin is an organ, not just the outside layer we can see, and it not only protects what is inside of us, but it acts as a pathway of excretion of waste from the body, if the usual channels of excretion — the bowels and/or the urinary system — are overloaded. The detoxification work of the liver is intricately linked to these processes too.

Course of action
The first place I always start when approaching the skin — which I wrote about in detail in *Beauty from the Inside Out* — is with a focus on the elimination and detoxification processes of the body. In Sarah's case, this involved dietary change, some additional nutrients, such as zinc and essential fatty acids, as well as a herbal medicine tonic designed for Sarah.

Outcome
It took two months for Sarah's skin to fully clear, but she said that, about 10 days after our initial consultation, she could tell she was on the right track as the redness came out of the pimples and fewer new ones started to form. What astonished Sarah was that she went down a size in her jeans over the two-month period of focusing on her skin. This was something she had wanted to do (and which was appropriate for her health status), but she hadn't had any results with things she had tried in the past, including counting the calories she was eating and those she was burning on an app on her phone.

You need to be healthy to lose weight. Sarah focused on her skin and got the desired outcome, but in the process she lost a jean-size.

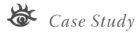 *Case Study*

Kerry's Story

Kerry was 58 when she came to see me. She said she couldn't lose weight no matter how much exercise she did and how little she ate. She had tried everything, she said.

While answering my zillion questions, Kerry said she had had her gallbladder removed after the birth of her second child, about 30 years before. She had also had a scan of her liver four years prior to now, and she had been told that she had a fatty liver. To my mind, she had many symptoms that demonstrated this as well. (See the "Liver" section for symptoms that your liver may need some support; but please note that these do not necessarily indicate a fatty liver, but may simply demonstrate that diet and lifestyle changes may be necessary to better support the liver.)

Course of action
I changed Kerry's diet and gave her some liver herbs, as well as a food-based greens powder. I asked her to get in touch if oil came away in a bowel motion, as, given that we were wanting to treat this, this would be a good sign. (Please note that if you notice oil in a bowel motion and it is unexpected, it is wise to see your GP.)

Outcome
On day eight, Kerry phoned to say that oil had come away with her bowel motion that morning. She felt fine and went to work as normal. Over the next three months, this continued — not with every bowel motion, but quite regularly — and Kerry kept a diary of any oil in her bowel motions, how she was feeling and what else she was observing.

Kerry was very focused on weight and was determined to remain that way. Her weight remained the same up until week seven, when it decreased; at the same time, she also noticed that a roll of fat underneath her bra line was significantly flatter. At the review appointment she made three months after the initial appointment, her whole face had altered and she was noticeably slimmer. Kerry said that she felt great and was sleeping better, and was nowhere near as frustrated with life as she had been. She said she had lost 6 kilograms, but they had all come off since week seven, which she found fascinating. She now only needed to keep eating real food, as her body had rid itself of at least some, if not all, of the fat that had been stored in the liver, and that had been interfering with Kerry's ability to lose body fat.

Stop dieting and counting calories. If you have to count something, count nutrients.

Dr Libby

The Foundation of Nourishment

I have included a chapter about digestion in each of my previous three paperbacks; a page of information about this topic even appears in my cookbooks. I have to include it here as well, because it is central to every aspect of health, including influencing what calories are worth, via the types of gut bacteria that inhabit our large intestine. If you have read my other books, feel free to skip this section, although it might be worth re-reading this material to help you really understand the concepts and then be able to apply them. No aspect of the calorie equation considers digestive system anomalies, and by not factoring it in this does us a disservice.

You may be someone who has intermittent challenges with your bowel. If so, you may notice that when your bowel is not behaving you either lose weight or gain weight, without focusing on weight or without your food and movement patterns changing. Let's firstly explore how the digestive system works.

The Digestive System

When making changes to optimize your health, including weight management, improving your digestion is a key place to start. We all know that it is best to build a house on a strong foundation, and building a robust digestive system is much the same. Gut issues are widespread, with one in five women in many Western countries reportedly suffering from irritable bowel syndrome (IBS). You only have to look at the amount of advertising targeted at improving gut health to see the prevalence of this problem. Improving digestion can have the most profound effect on your overall health and appearance. With simple, easy steps, you can experience radical changes.

It never ceases to amaze me how magnificent and how clever our bodies really are, and it astounds me how many processes go on inside the body without us having to give them any thought. Digestion is one of those processes, and it is central to every aspect of our well-being; it is the way we get all of the goodness out of our food, and the nourishment we get as a result of good digestion is an extraordinary gift without which we would not survive.

Digestion is intricate and complex, and yet relatively robust. And it is intimately connected to how you feel and function every single day, from your energy level to the fat you burn, from the texture and appearance of your skin to whether you have a bloated tummy, right down to your mood. Digestion is responsible for so much that goes on inside us. If it is a body system that gives you grief, if you are bloated most evenings, if you have intermittent diarrhoea and constipation, or if you get reflux, you can reach a point where you feel as though this is how life is always going to be. It must just be how you are. Perhaps you believe it is "in the family". Well, bowel challenges do *not* have to be your reality.

Digestion is the first place to start for amazing health. It can be a challenge to balance hormones, for example, if your digestion is the bane of your life. Likewise, if the gut is not working optimally, it will often show up in the skin, as the skin is just another pathway of elimination for the body. Some of the information in this section may make you grin or screw your face up ... it can be a challenge to find the right words to describe our stools. And some of the advice may at first seem obvious and too simple to make much of a difference. But reflect on your own eating habits and digestive system functions as you read on, and be ready to take your well-being to a new level.

> *I*t never ceases to amaze me how magnificent and how clever our bodies really are.

How the Digestive System Works

Digestion sustains us. It is the process of breaking down food so that we can absorb and utilize it for energy, and to maintain life. Food is simply broken down into smaller components. For example, proteins are broken down into amino acids, and it is through this breakdown of food, and our absorption of these smaller substances, that we are nourished.

The digestive system is made up of a digestive tract — a big, long tube (like a hose) — and numerous ancillary organs, including the liver, gallbladder and pancreas. The following illustration gives you an idea of what it looks like and how it works. The big, long tube begins at your mouth, moves down the oesophagus, then through a valve and into your stomach. The food then moves through a valve on the bottom side of the stomach and into the small intestine, through the small intestine and ileocaecal valve into the large intestine, and from there any waste is excreted out of the other end. When this process works well, you look and feel fantastic. When it is in any way impaired, the opposite can be true, and correcting it can change your life.

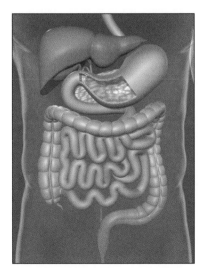

The human digestive system: The oesophagus enters the stomach (a cut-away section is shown above). The tube continues into the small intestine (the smooth tube above) and then into the large intestine (the indented tube section above). Finally, the waste is excreted. The liver is shown high on the left, the gallbladder is tucked in underneath the liver on the left, and the pancreas appears to sit behind the stomach pouch in the centre of the upper third of the image.

Supporting Digestion

While digestion usually takes place without your being aware of it, there are ways in which you can help the process be efficient. As digestion is about breaking food down to extract nutrients and expelling what is not needed, you can help the process by selecting what food you give it to work with, and by making the breaking-down process easier. The following are some ways you can support your digestive system.

Chew Your Food

Food enters the mouth and moves down the oesophagus into the stomach. But what do we do to our food before it reaches the stomach? We chew it — or, in some cases, inhale it! There are no more teeth beyond the mouth: we can't chew food once it has left our mouth. Yet so many people eat as though their oesophagus is lined with teeth. Many of us are in such a hurry with our meals, or we are so excited by the flavour of our food, that we might chew each mouthful four times if we are lucky. It is a case of chew, chew, chew, chew, mmmmm yum, next forkful in, chew, chew, oh gosh my mouth is so full, better swallow some food ... So we swallow some partially chewed food and some not-at-all-chewed food — and we do this day in, day out, year after year. And somehow we expect our stomach to cope. This alone can be the basis of digestive system problems, such as bloating, that appear further along the tract.

The stomach can get to a point where it doesn't like the rules by which you are playing anymore, and it finds it difficult to co-operate. So, slow down! Chew your food! If you are a food inhaler, try this: put food into your mouth, chew it really well, and then swallow it before you put the next mouthful in. I know that sounds simple, but try it. It can take an enormous amount of concentration for food inhalers to change their eating behaviours. Put your fork or spoon down between each mouthful if that helps. Engage in conversation between mouthfuls if you are eating with others. Savour the flavours, and the flavour combinations. Or think of your own technique to slow yourself down if you rush your food. You need to pay attention when you eat to *how* you eat.

Watch Portion Size

Now, back to the stomach, the first place food lands after you swallow it. Make a fist and observe its size. That is how big your stomach is without any food in it. Tiny, isn't it? So, think about what happens when you pile your plate high in the evening and swallow that big mountain of food. Your stomach has to stretch to accommodate it. And food sits in the stomach for a minimum of 30 minutes to allow the stomach acid and other digestive juices to keep breaking down the food.

Once your stomach gets used to being stretched, it expects it every day, and this stretching is the reason why, if you decide to eat less or go on a "diet", you tend to feel hungry after your meals for around four days, as it can take a few days for the nerve endings around your stomach pouch to shrink back. The nerves fire when they reach a certain stretching point, and then send a message to the brain to let you know you have eaten.

This is one of the numerous mechanisms we have that has the potential to tell us to stop eating, that we have had enough. The trouble is that, for some of us, the stomach is so used to being stretched that, by the time the nerves fire, we may have already over-eaten, started to feel lousy, and begun to berate ourselves.

The process described above is how carbohydrates let us know we have eaten. With fat and protein, however, as soon as we start to chew, messages are already being sent from the mouth to the satiety centre of the brain to let us know we are eating. These signals usually reach the brain within five minutes of chewing, while the stomach-stretch method can take more like 20 minutes. This explains why it is important to include fats and/or protein with each meal, as you are likely to eat less and be satisfied with less total food for that meal than if you simply ate carbohydrates on their own.

A rough guide to the amount of food we need to eat at each meal is approximately two fist-sized servings of concentrated food, such as proteins, fats and/or carbohydrates. You can, and need to, add to that as many water-based vegetables, such as green leafy vegies (non-starch vegetables and/or salad), as you like. Although greens have a high nutrient content, they are mostly water.

Wake Up Your Stomach Acid pH

Food arrives at the stomach after you chew and swallow it. The aroma of food, but particularly the chewing action itself, stimulates stomach acid production, which is an exceptionally important substance when it comes to great digestion. Stomach acid's role is to break food down. Imagine your food is a big, long string of circles, as shown in the first row of the illustration below. It is the job of the stomach acid to go chop, chop, chop, and break the circles apart into smaller bunches, as the second row illustrates.

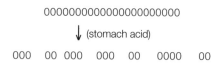

OOOOOOOOOOOOOOOOOOOOOOOO

↓ (stomach acid)

OOO   OO OOO   OOO   OO   OOOO   OO

Digestion: The action of stomach acid on whole foods breaks them down into their smaller components.

There are specific, ideal pH ranges for each tissue and fluid in the body. In scientific terms, pH refers to the concentration of hydrogen ions present, but you don't need to worry about that to understand this very important process.

pH is a measure of acidity or alkalinity. Its range is based on a scale of 0 to 14, with 0 being the acid end of the spectrum and 14 being the alkaline end; 7 is neutral. Every fluid, every tissue, every cell of your body has a pH at which it performs optimally. The optimal pH of stomach acid is around 1.9, which is so acidic that it would burn you if it touched your skin. But it doesn't burn you while it is nicely housed inside your stomach, as the cells that line the stomach itself not only produce stomach acid but are also designed to withstand the super-acidic conditions.

For many people though, the pH of the stomach acid is not acidic enough, and it may have a pH far greater than 1.9, which is not ideal for digestion. To be precise, animal proteins are optimally digested at a pH of 1.9, while starch is optimally digested at a pH of 2.1 which may not seem like much number-wise, but inside your body for some (not everyone) it can mean the difference between a flat abdomen and a bloated abdomen after a meal. A professor in the United States has been researching the pH of stomach acid in various groups of people who have been diagnosed with specific conditions, such as children with autism spectrum disorder (ASD). Many children with ASD have been found to have a stomach acid pH of around 4, far too high to effectively digest protein or starch.

Adults with reflux or indigestion tend to assume that the burning sensation they experience with heartburn means they are producing too much acid, when the opposite is usually true. They are usually not making enough stomach acid and/or the pH of it is too high. To understand this, remember the food-as-a-string-of-circles analogy and that stomach acid plays a vital role in breaking the circles apart. A pH that is much higher than 1.9 cannot effectively break the circles apart, and larger segments of, for example, seven circles in length may be the result. The body knows that if something seven circles in length continues along the digestive tract, it is not going to be able to further digest these partially broken-down circles. Rather than allowing that food to proceed down into the small intestine for the next part of its journey, the body regurgitates the food in an attempt to get rid of it, which is when you experience the acid burn. It "burns" you, because anything with a pH that is too acidic for the tissue to which it is exposed will create a burning sensation. When the acid is contained inside the stomach pouch, all is well; however, when it escapes out of this area, the lining of the oesophagus and the first part of the small intestine are not designed to cope with such acidic contents. Many people with reflux respond well to the stimulation of stomach acid and/or omitting problematic foods, and experience much fewer symptoms as a result.

As mentioned, stomach acid is stimulated by chewing and the aroma of food, as well as by the consumption of lemon juice and apple cider vinegar (ACV). The chewing action sends a message to the brain to send a message to the stomach to let it know that food is on its way. When we inhale our food, this doesn't happen. In the past, we took much longer to prepare our meals, and the slow-cooking processes generated an aroma of the upcoming meal, signalling the stomach that food was on its way.

Lemon juice and ACV physically stimulate the production of stomach acid. If you haven't consumed either of these before, it is best to initially dilute them and ideally consume them 5 to 20 minutes before breakfast (or all of your main meals if that appeals). For example, you might begin with half a teaspoon of ACV in as much water as you like. Over the coming days and weeks, you could gradually work up to having one tablespoon of ACV while you gradually decrease (or not) the amount of water. If you prefer lemon juice, start with the juice of half a lemon diluted to your tastes with *warm* water, and gradually work up to having the juice of a whole lemon in less warm water. If you use lemon, it can be a good idea to brush your teeth about 20 minutes after your meals to prevent any potential problems with tooth enamel in the future. Use these tips to wake up your stomach acid before you eat, as, without this area of the digestive system working optimally, it can have a significant impact not only locally, but further along the digestive system, and systemically on everything from energy to mood, from fat burning to restorative sleep.

The potential effect of drinking water with meals

We need the pH of our stomach acid to sit at around 1.9. Water has a pH of 7 (neutral pH) or above, depending on the mineral content — the higher the mineral content, the higher/more alkaline the pH. When you add a liquid with a pH of 7 or more to one with a pH of 1.9, what do you potentially do to the stomach acid? You dilute it. And we need all of the digestive fire we can muster to get the maximum nourishment out of our food and the best out of us. In my ideal world, we wouldn't drink water for 30 minutes on either side of eating.

You do not need to be concerned about the water content of food, nor do you need to focus on omitting all beverages at every meal. Simply aim to drink water between meals, not with meals. It can be a challenging habit to break. Set yourself a goal of not drinking with meals for one week, and then preferably keep the new habit going. Or add a squeeze of fresh lemon juice if you want water during your meal, but preferably not, particularly if you

> *We* need all of the digestive fire we can muster to get the maximum nourishment out of our food.

want to resolve gut challenges. Just cut it out for a week — one little week out of your very long life — and see if you feel any different.

Stimulate the pH Gradient of the Digestive System

Once food has been partially broken down in the stomach, it moves through the pyloric sphincter, a one-way valve leading into the duodenum, which is the beginning of the small intestine. In your body this valve is located in the middle, or just slightly on the left, of the chest, just below the bra line.

While food is in the stomach, messages are sent to the pancreas to secrete sodium bicarbonate, which has a highly alkaline pH, along with digestive enzymes. The bicarbonate is designed to protect the lining of the first part of the small intestine, while allowing digestion to continue. What is known as a "pH gradient" is established all the way along the digestive tract, and each region of the big long tube has an ideal pH. When the pH gradient is not established in the stomach — that is, when the pH is higher than ideal — digestion problems are likely further along the tract. These may be symptoms of the small or large intestine, such as bloating, pain or excessive wind. The absorption of nutrients may also be compromised. Insufficient pancreatic bicarbonate production may also cause digestive symptoms, such as a burning sensation underneath the stomach in the valve area described above. Pain in this area can also indicate that the gallbladder needs some support or investigation. It is best to consult with your health professional about this if you regularly feel discomfort in this area.

The best way to let the pancreas know that it needs to jump to action and produce bicarbonate and digestive enzymes is to have good stomach acid production at optimal pH. The digestive system runs off a cascade of signals from one organ or area to the next, via the brain. Use the suggested strategies, especially chewing food well, to stimulate the pancreas to fulfil its role.

There are occasions when I have suggested that clients use supplements of pancreatic enzymes, and this is appropriate if there is a genuine lack of digestive enzymes, rather than simply poor stomach acid conditions. I usually suggest the aforementioned strategies before trialling these supplements; however, when symptoms are severe, and once other causes have been ruled out, a gastroenterologist may measure pancreatic enzyme levels.

Promote Absorption

As food moves through the small bowel, digestive enzymes are secreted from the pancreas and the brush border, or lining, of the small intestine. The role of these enzymes is to continue what the stomach acid began, which is to continue to break down the food that has been eaten into its smallest, most basic components. It is in the small intestine where you absorb all of the goodness (ie, vitamins and minerals) out of your food. Think about that. All of the nutrients that keep you alive are drawn out of your food in the gut and move across into your blood so that your body can use those nutrients to do all of their life-sustaining jobs. The small intestine is where the nutrients in your food move from the tube that is your digestive tract into the blood, which is obviously a different set of tubes. This is how we are nourished, and it is how we stay alive.

Alcohol and vitamin B$_{12}$ are virtually the only substances you absorb directly out of your stomach into your blood, rather than via your small intestine. Alcohol tends to be in your blood within five minutes of consuming it, which is why you may get tipsy if you drink on an empty stomach.

Just because you eat something, though, doesn't mean you get all of the goodness out of it. If a food, for example, contains 10 milligrams of zinc, you don't necessarily absorb the whole 10 milligrams when you eat it. The absorption of nutrients is dependent on a whole host of factors, some of which have been discussed above. If you inhale your food, drink water with your meals, or have poor stomach acid production, for example, you may absorb very little of the goodness in your food. Nutrients are essential for life, and the *way* you are eating — let alone the foods you might be choosing — may be robbing you of some of the goodness your food provides, which can have an impact on every body system. Give yourself the best opportunity to absorb as much goodness out of your food as possible by applying the tips above. It may add energy to your years, and years to your life.

Address Niggling Pain

Many clients describe an on-again, off-again pain that hits them quite low down on the right-hand side of their abdomen. If you place your little finger on your right hip bone and use your thumb to find your navel, this pain tends to be located about halfway in between on that diagonal line. This is the *ileocaecal valve*, where the small intestine meets the large intestine. Many people have mistaken ileocaecal valve pain for appendicitis, as the appendix is located not far from this area. Always see a medical professional to diagnose your pain.

For many, pain begins in this area after food poisoning or a stomach bug (infection), after travelling, usually overseas, or camping. When you had the bug, you might have had bouts of diarrhoea. Even though the obvious symptoms of the causative infection have long since gone, it is as though the nasty little critters that caused the original upset tummy have taken up residence in the valve. Or perhaps they have changed its function or led to other bacteria inhabiting this area that don't belong there.

To remedy this pain, there are numerous options to try. One is to release the reflex connected to this valve by rubbing the area with your fingertips 20 times in an anticlockwise circular motion with reasonable pressure, not so it hurts you but also not with super-soft fingers. Another option is to use anti-parasitic herbs, such as Chinese wormwood and Black walnut, every day for four to eight weeks, before each main meal, under the guidance of a health professional. The other potential remedy is one of my favourite substances on Earth: Lugol's iodine. The liquid of potassium iodide is not only a source of iodine, which is necessary for so many body functions, but it acts as a potent anti-parasitic agent that seems to help clear nasty critters from this important valve. It is possible to overdose on iodine, though, so it is best to check your dosage with a health professional to make sure you take the dose that is right for you.

Promote Good Gut Bacteria

Once the food gets to the large intestine, can you guess what lives there? Bacteria. On average, an adult will have 3–4 kilograms of bacteria living in their colon. So, just as an aside, every time you weigh yourself remember that three to four of the kilos you see in that number on the scales is made up of gut bacteria that are essential for life; another reason why it is crazy that we weigh ourselves.

Some of the bacteria in your large bowel (colon) are good guys, and some are bad guys. You want more good guys than bad guys. The role of the gut bacteria is to ferment whatever you give them. To come back to the circle concept of food illustrated previously, gut bugs love it when you give them something that is one or even two circles in size. They know what to do with that. But if a previous digestive process was not completed sufficiently, the bacteria in your colon may be presented with fragments of food that are five or even seven circles in size, and all they know to do with such fragments of food is ferment it.

What word springs to mind when you think of fermentation? I love asking this question at my seminars, as the answers usually amuse me as well as the audience. People will often say "beer", "wine", "sauerkraut"! But usually I eventually get the answer I am after, which is gas. Fermentation involves bacterial action on a food source, and the subsequent production of gas. Some gases are essential to the health of the cells that line our gut, while others seem to irritate the gut and give us a bloated, uncomfortable stomach as the day progresses, whether we have eaten in a healthy way or not. These unfriendly gases also add a load to the liver, so they could be deemed a "problematic substance" for the body; an additional liver-loader that we don't need in a world with too many of these already.

The trouble with a bloated stomach for many women, in particular, is that it messes with their brain. When they look down and see a swollen tummy, something inside immediately communicates to every cell of their body that they have gained weight, whether they consciously think this thought or not. Many of my clients go up a size around the waist as the day progresses, even though they feel they have eaten with their health in mind. This can add a layer of stress to a woman's life that they just don't need or understand. It is especially stressful because they can't fathom why it is happening. Sometimes it is the foods and drinks you are choosing. Sometimes it is the bugs that live in your colon. Sometimes it is because of poor digestion further up the process, such as insufficient stomach acid. In traditional Chinese medicine (TCM), bloating is often considered a spleen and/or liver picture, and a TCM practitioner is likely to use acupuncture and/or herbs to support the spleen and liver. Sometimes bloating is due to too much coffee, or from stress and living on adrenalin, in what I have come to call "the red zone".

Address Stress

Poor digestion can be due to stress or, more precisely, adrenalin, a stress hormone. The perception of stress or real stress drives the body to make adrenalin, and it diverts the blood supply away from digestive processes and concentrates the blood in your periphery, your arms and legs, allowing you to escape from the danger you are supposedly in. If blood were still concentrated on the digestive system, there is a risk you would be distracted by food or hunger, thus putting your survival at risk. These concepts are explored in detail in the section that discusses stress hormones and their impact on the calories you consume.

Ensure Complete Bowel Evacuation

In dealing with clients one-on-one, I have had to work out ways to extract information from people using words that accurately describe what is going on for that person. Many years ago, one of the questions I originally found difficult to phrase was around how empty someone felt after they had used their bowels. I tried to dream up ways to phrase this question so that it would not make clients feel uncomfortable, but also so that I could gain greater insight into how their bowel was functioning. As with many things, a client turned out to have the answer. While asking him about his bowel habits, he said, "You know what? My greatest discomfort comes from incomplete evacuation." There they were. The words I needed. So, early on in my consultation work with people, I started asking about feelings of incomplete evacuation. For some, it is not an issue at all. They have no idea what I am talking about when I mention it. For others, they are so excited that someone has finally given them the words to describe such frustrating discomfort. They wouldn't answer "yes" if I asked them if they were constipated, as they may use their bowels every day. It is just that when they do go to the toilet, they feel like there is more to come but it doesn't eventuate and evacuate.

This feeling can be the result of numerous scenarios. It may be insufficient digestive processes as outlined previously. It may be inadequate production of digestive enzymes due to poor signalling, or a damaged or inflamed brush border. It may be a food allergy or intolerance. It could be undiagnosed coeliac disease. It could be related to fibre or dehydration. It can be stress hormones causing the muscles surrounding the bowel to contract and hold onto waste. It may be a magnesium deficiency not allowing the walls of the bowel to relax and allow the thorough passage of waste. Or the thyroid gland may not be working optimally. TCM teaches us that it is insufficient spleen and/or liver energy ... The list of scenarios is almost endless, but finding those specific for you can change your health, your waistline and the way you experience life.

Dietary change: dietary trials
One option to improve this challenge is to have a health professional help you get to the heart of it and remedy the situation. You might increase your green vegetable intake and decrease the processed foods in your diet for a week, and see if that makes a difference, especially given that green vegetables are good sources of magnesium, water and fibre, amongst other things. Plus, in eliminating processed foods for this trial period, you will be missing out on artificial substances such as preservatives and colourings, and this alone may make a difference.

You may be suspicious that a food or a group of foods is causing this feeling for you, but because you love this food you are reluctant to remove it. I cannot encourage you enough to remove suspicious food from your diet for a *trial* period of two weeks (four is even better). Two little weeks out of your very long life — an expression I use regularly with clients to highlight the relatively short time period necessary to potentially offer enormous insight into their health challenges. For some, however, a longer trial of three months is necessary, best done with the guidance of a health professional. You may get an answer to your challenge over the trial period; if not, you can relax and thoroughly enjoy this food without silently worrying. But I can hear you already asking: "What if it works?

What does that mean? Will I never eat that food again?" My answer is always that it is your choice.

I have witnessed people be resistant to dietary change, but after a time feel so different, so much better, that they have no desire to ever go back to the way they used to eat. I have met others who, even though they may feel better, still miss a food terribly. In the latter scenario, I suggest to them after the trial that it is a good thing that now they know the culprit. It is no longer a mystery to them why they feel this way. Then they are in control. Unless the problem is a true allergy, I find that when people are strong — meaning when they are very robust from a digestion perspective — their gut will tolerate this food better than if they are stressed. Either way, once you know, you are in control and it is your choice. Unless the food is a true allergy for you, your tolerance of it may change and improve over time, especially with a focus on gut healing and stress management. Don't think that because it hurts you today it always will. Your body changes and renews itself constantly. Just know there is a reason for your symptom(s). It is simply a matter of finding your answers.

Softening waste

One of the reasons I am so concerned with bowel evacuation is that, if this process is inefficient, waste can remain inside the bowel for too long. While it is there, it is fermenting. This can give the liver additional and unnecessary toxins to process, as well as "suffocate" the cells that line the colon. No one has studied the impact of this on the way energy (ie, calories) is used in your body.

The waste can also dry out and harden, sticking itself to the lining of the bowel wall, narrowing the tube through which the new waste can flow. If you have ever seen soil in the middle of a drought — cracked, dried-out and unable to absorb a brief shower of rain — that is the way hardened faeces can behave in your colon.

If this scenario occurs, waste can move only through the middle of this newly formed, faeces-lined tube, and the efficiency of waste elimination is decreased. The old, hard, compacted faecal matter remains. When the cells that line the bowel are coated with hard faeces, they are unable to "breathe", and a process that was once described in medical textbooks as *auto-intoxication* can ensue. To remedy this, chamomile is one of the best things you can take. Either drink plenty of chamomile tea, take capsules, or have the medicinal herb prescribed and have it with each meal. Once the waste has dried out, it is difficult to rehydrate it so that it can move through and be excreted. Chamomile softens the waste and helps the bowel wall relax.

Colonics

Another potential remedy is one about which many people have very strong opinions: colon hydrotherapy, or colonics. This process involves a tube being inserted into a person's rectum through which warm or cool water gently flows. This allows the hardened faecal matter to soften, like heavy, consistent rain on dried-out soil, allowing the large bowel to empty fully, often getting rid of built-up waste that may have been there for a very long time. I have had clients tell me that the waste they excreted during their first colonic was black, inferring that it may have been there for many years, interfering with healthy bowel function. I had a lady once tell me she saw popcorn in the viewing pipe during her colonic — and she knew that the last time she had eaten popcorn was at the movies over six months beforehand!

Colonics polarize people. The idea either appeals to you or it doesn't. There seems to be no middle ground with people's love or dislike of colon hydrotherapy. I encourage you, though, not to lose sight of the effect that trends have had on medicine. Up until the early 1900s, colonics were accepted as part of general medicine. Doctors understood the importance of good bowel evacuation, and considered colonics to be a normal treatment method for a host of health conditions, not just bowel issues. Coffee enemas were actually cited in the *Merck Manual for Doctors* for liver detoxification until 1972.

With a well-functioning bowel, an enormous load is taken off not only the digestive system but also the liver, one of the organs primarily responsible for cleansing our body. Help prevent bowel cancer by ensuring efficient bowel evacuation using methods that suit you. Always seek advice from a health professional before undertaking colon hydrotherapy, if that option appeals to you.

Gut Integrity and Opioid Effects

An additional concept within digestive health is not only fascinating but has wide-ranging effects on how we feel and function, including gut transit time (ie, how quickly food moves through the digestive system), mood, concentration and, potentially, food addictions. This concept is known as the *opioid excess theory*.

Gut Integrity

The cells that line a healthy small intestine look like a row of bricks with finger-like projections (called *villi*), neatly stacked side-by-side as demonstrated in the picture below.

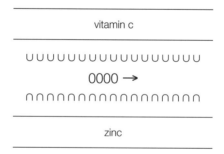

A healthy gut: Food (represented here by the circles) travelling through a healthy mature intestine moves straight ahead. Only nutrients (for example, vitamin C and zinc) enter the blood vessels that closely follow the intestines.

In a healthy gut, only the tiny nutrients (vitamins and minerals) diffuse (move) through the gut wall into the blood, and this is the precious process through which we are nourished and stay alive. However, the cells that line the gut can come apart, as if the bricks have gaps between them, as illustrated below. This is also how our gut is when we are born.

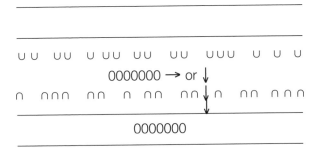

A "leaky" gut: Food (represented here by the circles) travels through an immature gut or a "leaky" intestine. Microscopic, poorly digested fragments of food can escape out of the gut and enter the blood.

When we are born, the cells that line our digestive system are a distance apart, which is why we can't feed all foods to newborns; foods must be gradually introduced to a child over time as the gut matures, to prevent allergies developing. The gut is immature when we are born, and it slowly matures from birth until reaching full maturity somewhere between the ages of two and five, depending on the individual child and their health and life experiences in the early years. Sadly, for some this maturation process may be stunted by constant ill health until gut health is addressed.

The cells that line the gut can, however, also come apart during adulthood as a result of a gastrointestinal infection or stress. The chronic production of stress hormones can compromise the integrity of the gut cells and signal to them that they need to move further apart so that more nutrition can get through to the blood, as nutrient requirements increase during times of stress. Everything about us is geared for survival.

When food travels through a gut with good cell-lining integrity, it can only go straight ahead. However, if it travels through a gut in which the cells have come apart, it may go straight ahead or it may move out of the gut and into the blood. Fragments of food are not intended to enter the blood.

Nutrients — the vitamins and minerals from food — are. So if fragments of food enter the blood stream, the immune system, which is what protects you from infection, thinks that the food fragment is a germ and it mounts an immune response against it. This is one way adults develop food sensitivities.

Poor gut integrity is also described as "leaky gut". Once you were able to eat anything without a problem, and now certain foods seem to cause you grief. This process can be healed by minimizing irritation to the gut lining, which can mean avoiding some foods or ingredients for a period of time, while also working on gut integrity. Aloe vera juice to start the day can also assist an irritated gut. Again, no one has studied the impact of energy (ie, calorie) intake on body shape and size when they have increased gut permeability. Given fragments of food that are too large end up in the blood supply in a leaky gut state, I consider this to be extra "stress" on the body, or perhaps an addition to the toxin load. And, as you will see throughout the pages of this book, both of these factors potentially influence your calorie needs and whether you will burn body fat or store it.

> Leaky gut can be healed by minimizing irritation to the gut lining, which can mean avoiding some foods or ingredients for a period of time, while also working on gut integrity.

Often people are able to tolerate the foods that cause them grief once we have worked out why they have leaky gut symptoms in the first place. Did the problem begin as a result of stress or an infection? The power to heal the symptoms is always in the "why".

The Opioid Effect

The blood supply into which the food fragments flow is the same blood supply that goes to your brain. Humans have what is known as the blood–brain barrier, a semi-permeable layer separating the peripheral blood supply from that of the brain. The blood–brain barrier was always considered to be a highly selective membrane that only allowed substances into the brain that would be of benefit. However, research has now shown that this is not the case. In cases where gut permeability is increased, the blood–brain barrier is often suspected of having the same increased permeability.

If we could see the food fragments, their structure is very similar to that of opioids. Opioids are substances that help humans feel good. They also help modulate pain. We have our own natural feel-good hormones, endorphins, which have an opioid-based structure. In our brain and in our gut, we have what are called opioid receptors. To review: just because your body makes a substance (ie, a chemical messenger or hormone), that doesn't mean you necessarily get the effects of that substance. For you to get the effect generated by that hormone, the substance must bind to a receptor, just like a lock and a key fitting together. In this case, when we make endorphins and they bind to the opioid receptors, we feel pleasure. Heroin and morphine are opioids, and they, too, bind to the opioid receptors in the brain. Anything that gives a human pleasure has the potential to be addictive, hence the aforementioned drugs. You can also see from this example how someone might become addicted to exercise. Activity tends to generate endorphins. So whenever you partake in or experience something that gives you pleasure — like a sunset, a spin class, a tennis game, or a child's laughter — you make endorphins which bind to opioid receptors, and you feel pleasure.

How does this relate to food, body fat and over-eating? Some of the fragments of food that can escape out of a leaky gut into the blood stream can also have an opioid structure. These include beta-casomorphine and gluteomorphine. They are partially digested fragments of casein (a major protein in cow's milk products) and gluten (a major protein in wheat, rye, barley, oats and triticale). Just like endorphins, these opioids from food also have the capacity to bind to the opioid receptors in the brain and very subtly make us feel good. The effect is not usually noticed as an enormous boost in mood, but the person will often feel as though they can't live without this food, and they will feel as though they *have* to eat it in some form daily or even at every meal. Sometimes they start eating it and they can't stop, although this can be due to numerous reasons, not just an opioid effect.

I have seen this to be the case with countless clients. If a patient has a set of symptoms that warrants them omitting a food from their diet for a trial period to see if it will make a difference, some people have no problem. There is no resistance. Others will beg me not to take them off a food for a trial, yet they are seeing me because they want results, and all I am asking is four measly weeks of omitting a particular food that may just give them the answer to some of their health concerns! I am not judging someone who responds in this way; I am simply pointing out to you that the power food can have over an individual can be just like an addiction. An individual's connection to a certain food is often highly emotional, and also potentially physical, through this opioid mechanism.

Food was never intended to fill these roles for humans. However, on a physical level, where there is a leaky gut, it is possible that the opioid effect, which some foods have the potential to create, might be one of the factors behind food addictions, and, hence for some, over-eating or eating and not feeling like you can stop. This is an area that deserves much more research, time and money, as the opioid excess theory may be involved in numerous health conditions as well as obesity. Much research has already been done in relation to children with autism and adults with schizophrenia, where these *exorphins* (opioids from an exogenous source — that is, consumed rather than made by the body) have been found to play a role in the expression of symptoms of these conditions.

Food not only has the capacity to affect our sleep, skin, body shape and size, but also our mood. Our digestion of some foods may also be incomplete, leading to the generation of an opioid effect and addiction to particular foods. If you suspect this process is going on for you, omit all sources of that dietary component (eg, gluten and/or casein) for a trial period of four weeks. The first four to seven days will be the most difficult, but persevere. The results may be enormously worth it. If you do omit significant dietary components from your diet for extended periods (beyond four weeks), it is important to consult a health professional to make sure you do not miss out on any nutrients essential for your health.

Support the Spleen — the TCM Perspective

The spleen rules digestion in traditional Chinese medicine (TCM). In TCM, each organ is considered to have its own vital energy, as well as there being whole-body energy. If spleen energy is down, you will feel your usual hunger for meals, but as soon as you eat even a small amount, you will feel full and possibly bloated. Your short-term memory is likely to not be what it once was, and you may possibly feel like you eat like a bird yet your weight continues to escalate. You can eat and exercise with a real commitment, but if spleen energy is low, from a TCM perspective, you won't feel like your best self, and you will likely feel that, no matter what you do, you can't lose weight.

Stimulating spleen energy can make a real difference. Acupuncture will do this, as will bitter herbs. Warming foods (referring to the unique properties foods have, according to TCM, as well as temperature) also help, as can adding warming spices, such as ginger, cumin and turmeric, to dishes. Spleen energy can also become low from "overthinking". The busy mind, relentlessly thinking of the next thing you need to do, takes energy away from the vital process of digestion every day, according to TCM principles. The spleen may also lose some of its strength if liver or kidney energy is overbearing or low. (The adrenals, which produce stress hormones (as well as other hormones), sit on top of the kidneys.) Working with a wonderful TCM practitioner can also help you heal your gut, which in turn helps every aspect of your well-being, including how your clothes fit.

Consider Food Combining

Food combining can be a wonderful approach to eating that can enhance digestion, energy, vitality, and fat loss, and it can be a great way to combat a bloated tummy. It involves a few simple principles, including eating animal protein separately from starchy carbohydrates. In practice, that means no meat and potatoes on the same plate. It means that if you eat meat, chicken or fish, you eat it with high-water vegetables and no starchy vegetables, such as potato, sweet potato, pumpkin and corn, or any other starchy foods, such as pasta, bread or rice. If you eat vegetable protein, such as one of the many types of lentils, chickpeas or beans, then, using the food-combining principles, you do not eat meat with these foods, but instead any vegetable at all, including starchy ones if they appeal. If you feel like eating rice, then with food combining it needs to be a vegetarian meal. Oils and other foods rich in fats, including avocado, can be eaten with either animal-based meals or starch-based meals.

Another principle of food combining is that fruit is only consumed as your first meal and not again during the day. For some, instead of digesting it, it ferments, which can lead to a range of gut symptoms. You are also encouraged to omit all refined sugar and processed foods, as the main goal of food combining is to support the health of your blood, given it does all of the nutrient-dissemination work within the body.

I know people who live by the concept of food combining and feel spectacular. They are slim and find it effortless to maintain this, whether they regularly eat 2000 calories one day and 3000 calories another day, despite the Harris–Benedict Equation suggesting they can only eat 1600 calories per day for weight maintenance. For others, for whom food combining seems extreme, but who still want to try it, I suggest they apply the *zigzag principle*. This means that most of the time they follow food-combining principles (zig), while one day a week, or two to three meals a week, they relax the principles and they zag. This approach is more sustainable for some; you are still able to dine out and enjoy all foods, whatever combination arrives on your plate, but just not every day. Remember, it is what you do every day that impacts on your health, not what you do sometimes. It is important to note that this latter statement is *not* applicable to true food allergies — they must be strictly omitted from the diet.

Food combining is a structured way of eating that allows some individuals to thrive. I have seen this approach to diet truly change people's lives. For others, eating this way might take every aspect of joy out of their life. If this is the case for you, then focusing on food combining is not for you right now, or perhaps the zigzag concept might appeal. I am certainly not prescribing this for you. I simply want to offer you options to help you experience your best health and a new way of looking at how you fuel your body in a way that serves you.

Why Eat Real Food?

Scientists have created a tiny camera that sits inside a capsule (not unlike a dietary supplement capsule), which research participants swallow, thereby providing about 16 hours of footage from inside the digestive system. The researchers gave one group a real food meal, where they made noodles from scratch, from flour and water, and served it in a broth made from water, salt and vegetables. The other group was given a ready-meal bought from the supermarket: ramen noodles with 15 different ingredients on the label, along with a blue "sports" drink. After four hours, the camera footage showed that those in the real food group had only tiny, white pieces of fluff remaining in their digestive tract; the food was well broken down. For those in the bought-food group four hours after ingestion, you could still see the teeth marks in the noodles where the participants had bitten into them. There were still long strings of noodles remaining

> *R*emember, it is what you do every day that impacts on your health, not what you do sometimes.

intact four hours after eating. In addition to this, the noodles and part of the lining of the intestine had been dyed blue from the drink. This is the result of the dye in the drink being petroleum-based, and humans have no capability to break down petrol.

> *You don't have to lose weight to be healthy — you have to be healthy to lose weight.*

Eat real food. Your body has the equipment (ie, digestive enzymes) to break it down and provide you with the nourishment your body needs to function optimally. That includes weight loss. You don't have to lose weight to be healthy — you have to be healthy to lose weight.

Remember ...

Digestion is central and essential to every process in our body, which is why, when exploring the way the body uses calories, it is the base from which we build. As around 80% of your immune system lines your gut, when gut function is impaired it can have a significant impact on the immune system, with more and more research suggesting that this is where some autoimmune conditions originate.

So, whether your focus is optimizing your health and well-being, and/or improving a challenging or diseased gut, body fat management, or resolving congested skin, understanding your digestive system is a crucial step in your understanding of the calorie fallacy.

❖ The Foundation of Nourishment In Short ...

Your digestive system is the gateway for nutrients into your body, and it is nutrients that keep us alive. They are also essential for weight loss. Just because you eat a nutrient, doesn't mean you get it, though, as the absorption of nutrients can be compromised for many reasons.

Optimal digestion is also critical for healthy elimination, which is essential for the excretion of waste from the body. If waste accumulates, it can pose an additional load for the liver, also interfering with the effective burning of body fat as a fuel (explained in the "Liver" section). If the digestive system processes go awry early on during digestion, then partially digested food, instead of well digested food, can end up in the large intestine. As the bacteria that live there only know to ferment whatever is given to them, receiving partially digested food can lead to the production of excessive gaseous compounds, which can in turn lead to increased gut permeability and an increased load on the liver. Furthermore, if partially digested food fragments are created from poor digestion and the gut is leaky, these partially digested food fragments can end up crossing over into the blood, hyper-stimulating the immune system. They can cross the blood–brain barrier, impacting aspects of neuronal firing and leading people to feel addicted to specific foods.

Hence, chewing food well, eating slowly, and stimulating stomach acid production with apple cider vinegar or lemon juice in warm water, can all be highly beneficial ways to begin to positively help the digestive system.

Eat real food. Remember the experiments done with camera inside a capsule and the footage and insights that generated. Your body has the equipment (ie, digestive enzymes) to break it down and provide you with the nourishment your body needs to function optimally. That includes weight loss. You don't have to lose weight to be healthy — you have to be healthy to lose weight.

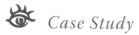

Case Study

Anne's Story

Sixty-three-year-old Anne came to see me, very despondent about her health and body. She had been a high-school home economics teacher and believed herself to have excellent nutrition knowledge and tremendous willpower. She had applied the Harris–Benedict Equation to calculate her energy requirements at the age of 30, and she had adapted it every five years as her age changed. She followed the dietary pyramid, eating low-fat dairy products and plenty of complex carbohydrates, such as wholegrain bread and wholegrain cereals. She had good muscle mass from sport she had played for much of her life, as well as from going to her supervised gym. She had come to see me as she was perplexed about what had happened with her health over the past two and a half years, since a trip to Turkey. During her time away she had had what she thought was food poisoning, where she had vomited for three days and had severe diarrhoea for three weeks. She had had to cut her trip short as she was so unwell.

On her return, the diarrhoea stopped but her bowels, even over two years later, were still erratic, and her GP had diagnosed IBS. She also had low iron, which she couldn't understand, as she ate good amounts of iron-rich foods and she was no longer menstruating. Her weight had also increased by 12 kilograms, even though she had returned to her strict calorie counting and exercise regime. Anne said she felt tired no matter how much sleep she had, and her hair was falling out. But she was also very concerned about her weight.

Diagnosis

As I had seen similar scenarios in plenty of previous patients, I was suspicious that the infection she had picked up on her travels had changed her gut bacteria profile. I was also suspicious that she may have undiagnosed coeliac disease, and I felt that this was worth initially exploring with a blood test, before I suggested any dietary change.

Anne was confirmed by blood test and then by small bowel biopsy to have coeliac disease. Whether she had had it longer than the bowel symptoms, we will never know. There is a strong chance that it was triggered by the infective event.

Course of action

I placed Anne on a gluten-free diet made from real, whole foods, not processed gluten-free foods.

Outcome

After nine months, not only did Anne feel "just wonderful", but her bowel motions were now daily and the stools well formed, her iron levels had replenished, and she had lost 14 kilograms. Anne reported to me that she was astonished by all that had unfolded, including that, based on her calculations, she was now eating on average 2500 calories per day, 50% of which were coming from fat, 20% from protein and 30% from carbohydrates. This was 850 calories more than she had eaten for much of her earlier adult life. She said, too, that having read one of my books, she had switched two of her other exercise sessions to yoga, and that was all the exercise she was doing now, along with a walk twice a week with a friend. She said that now, while her "calorie equation" was greatly in favour of eating too much and weight gain, her weight was stable and in a great place. She had lost 14 kilograms, when she had only gained 12 kilograms at the time she started her gluten-free, real food way of eating, and clearly this new pattern of eating was doing something wonderful for her health, as she felt vibrant and happy again.

*C*hange begins when you start acting like the person
you want to become.

Dr Libby

Feed the Good Bugs

In 2006, research conducted by scientists in the United States showed that what calories are worth to your body is influenced by the gut bacteria inhabiting your large intestine. Yet we never hear about this. For so many reasons, this one included, gut health is central to our overall well-being.

The bacterial species in the gut is an area in which I have had intense interest since starting my PhD, part of which involved analyzing faeces samples from children with autism spectrum disorder (ASD). Not really something to discuss at a dinner party!

One of the concepts my research taught me was that the way we eat is one of the factors that influence the species of gut bacteria that inhabit our colon. These bacteria eat and produce waste just as a human does. The pH of each portion of the colon is also a significant contributor to which species of gut bacteria are able to survive in a particular region. pH is influenced by a host of factors, including the metabolic by-products the bacteria themselves make, such as lactic acid.

Bacteroidetes and Firmicutes

Let's explore the influence gut bacteria have over the effect of calories on our body. The very clever research from the mid-2000s scientifically demonstrated what I had observed in my clients, and what countless clients already felt to be true: that is, there seem to be times in our lives when calories behave as though they are worth more to our body than at others.

The research initially took two groups of genetically identical mice with sterile guts; that is, there were no bacteria inhabiting their intestines. The researchers inoculated one group with a range of bacterial phylum that broadly fit under the name *Firmicutes*, while the other species were inoculated with *Bacteroidetes*. Both groups of mice were given an identical number of calories from identical food sources. The group that received the *Bacteroidetes* species remained the same weight and size, while the *Firmicutes* group gained weight. The mice looked "puffy" and "swollen" in the images presented in the scientific paper. This is the first research that showed that the types of gut bacteria present in the large bowel may influence the value of calories.

The results of this work went on to be replicated in humans. This study found that people categorized as obese for the purpose of the research had significantly fewer *Bacteroidetes* in their bowel than lean people in the study. Lean people had a dominance of *Bacteroidetes*. The 10 trillion to 100 trillion microorganisms that populate our adult intestines benefit us in a number of ways. One benefit is that they allow us to extract calories from otherwise indigestible common polysaccharides (carbohydrates) in our diet. This benefit occurs because components of the microbiota are able to adaptively deploy a large array of enzymes such as glycoside hydrolases and polysaccharide lysases that we do not encode in our genome. Furthermore, studies using germ-free and colonized normal and knockout mice fed a standard, polysaccharide-rich rodent-chow diet indicate that this mutualistic host-microbe relationship allows the extracted energy to be stored in fat cells through a pathway that involves microbial regulation of fat storage enzymes. Microbial fermentation of dietary polysaccharides to monosaccharides (single sugars) and short-chain fatty acids

> One of the concepts my research taught me was that the way we eat is one of the factors that influence the species of gut bacteria that inhabit our colon.

in the distal gut and their subsequent absorption stimulate the new (*de novo*) synthesis of triglycerides in the liver, potentially another mechanism contributing to non-alcoholic fatty liver disease.

Are you one of those people who feels like you only have to look at food for it to end up sticking to you? Do you notice what the people around you eat, and then wonder how you can be the size you are when you feel as though you eat like a bird? Do you feel that the way you eat is not reflected in your size? Well, there may be numerous factors at play in this scenario, such as elevated cortisol, oestrogen dominance, liver congestion, or excess calories (for meeting physical or emotional needs). At this stage, I simply want you to understand that the species of bacteria in your large bowel can also play a role.

When I ask people to change their diets for a period of time, usually four weeks initially, one of the questions in my head is how do I alter this person's gut bacterial profile so that their overall health improves, their energy improves, their appetite changes (if they over-eat in the first place), and their clothes get looser? The first step is to starve the "bad" bugs.

Just like humans, gut bacteria have food preferences, and they have specific nutritional requirements. Guess what they thrive on? Sugars! Now you have the biggest reason ever to eliminate refined sugars, in particular, from your diet for a minimum of four weeks. Not just reduce it. Eliminate it. You must frame it in your head as four tiny weeks out of your very long life. This small chunk of time may begin to give you an enormous health answer. If it feels overwhelming, perhaps take a leaf out of one of my client's book.

Nicole's Story

A client, Nicole, who began seeing me when she was 140 kilograms (she volunteered to share her weight; I didn't weigh her) taught me a way she found very effective to eliminate refined sugar from her diet. After hearing me speak at a seminar, she identified sugar as her biggest challenge. Cutting sugar back, let alone cutting it out completely, overwhelmed her. I bark on and on about the enormous importance of greens (green vegetables, especially green leaves), and so instead of starting by cutting out sugar Nicole simply focused on eating more greens. Within four weeks, she no longer even wanted sugar. Her words to me were "it tastes terrible, and I feel like I'm poisoning myself".

Extreme perhaps, but you get the message. Sugar tastes bad after a while of eating a lot of green foods, because greens are bitter, which makes the sugar taste sickeningly sweet by contrast. So increase your greens, and watch the sugar fall away, or utilize the increase in dietary fat from whole food sources as discussed in another section as a way of eliminating refined sugars.

Gut bugs don't just play a direct role in what calories are worth to your body though. They do this indirectly as well. Good gut bugs help support a healthy immune system; they support detoxification, particularly of heavy metals, which (to keep this simple) we are exposed to every day just through the number of cars on the road and/or via cigarette smoke, directly or passively.

Irritable Bowel Syndrome (IBS)

While I am presenting information about gut bacteria, I want to touch on irritable bowel syndrome (IBS), as one in five women in Australia and New Zealand is now affected by IBS. It is common, but it is not normal, and it doesn't have to be this way. Food is not supposed to bloat you.

The common symptoms of IBS include:

 # abdominal pain or cramping that is often relieved by passing wind or faeces

 # alternating diarrhoea and constipation

 # a sensation that the bowels are not fully emptied after passing a motion

 # abdominal bloating

 # mucous present in the stools

 # nausea.

Getting to the heart of why someone is experiencing IBS is critical, as the road into any condition is the road that needs to be taken out. In other words, if gluten is the basis for the IBS, then no amount of probiotics will resolve it. If the IBS is due to stress hormone production, then dietary change may not make a difference. Often, however, a number of strategies are required to resolve it, as you will see in a moment.

One of my concerns about ongoing, long-term IBS is the consequences for the liver. Some products of fermentation in the gut fuel the cells that line the gut, while others have to be shunted to the liver for detoxification. However, as you already understand, the liver has a huge amount on its plate in this day and age, and, when it can't keep up with the load, the "leftovers" are stored in the fatty tissues of the body. Resolving gut health challenges, including the profile of bacteria that inhabit the large intestine, is critical for appropriate utilization of calories, as well as feeling great. And none of this is considered in the calorie equation.

A bloated stomach can also mess with psychology, par-ticularly a female one. Regardless of your physical size, if you look down and see a bloated stomach, feelings of tension, disappointment, frustration or self-criticism can arise. You may have eaten what you consider to be incredibly healthy food that day, you may have exercised, and you may distinctly recall on waking that morning that your tummy was comfortable. Now it looks like you have swallowed a football. Logic tends to disappear at this point. If it could rear its head, logic would tell you that it is not possible to gain a football's worth of fat in a day and that your tummy is simply bloated, so calm down, things will be OK again in the morning, and it would be good to get to the bottom of your bloatedness. But the potential for that train of thought left the building the moment your brain saw your protruding tummy.

Even if you didn't eat nourishing food that day and you sat on your bottom for most of it, if you look down at the end of the day and see that your tummy has expanded, the psyche, especially the female one, either withdraws into themselves, is suddenly in a lousy mood, starts over-reacting to situations, gets teary at the drop of a hat, or thinks "what the heck" and eats the pantry empty! Some people will be aware of what led to their change in mood. Most are not. And it is worse for those who have been making conscious efforts with food and movement. The people who have eaten poorly that day still feel down about themselves, but they follow that flat feeling with thoughts that drive more lousy feelings, such as, "Well what did you expect? You ate biscuits when you said you weren't going to. You're so hopeless, you have no willpower, you'll *never* change." Hardly uplifting sentiments!

One of the biochemical factors that can contribute to the body getting the message that it needs to store fat in this scenario is via cortisol, the chronic stress hormone. Cortisol slows your metabolic rate, so, even if your food intake and movement have not altered, cortisol is catabolic, and breaks your muscles down. Hence, it slows metabolism, and clothes will typically get tighter. That's not due to calories. Your equation in this scenario has not changed. This is the result of the information being communicated to your body that it needs to store fat because, probably amongst other stresses in your life, you stressed out at your bloated tummy.

There are numerous issues to raise here to assist you to begin to get resolution from IBS, and potentially your gut bacteria profile. Some are physical, whereas others are emotional. Let's examine why your tummy keeps bloating. Ask yourself:

- Is it related to your menstrual cycle only?

- Does it only happen after you eat lunch? If so, what are you eating for lunch?

- Does your tummy bloat only after afternoon tea? What are you choosing for afternoon tea?

- Is it worse when you are stressed? Did it begin only after you went through a great deal of change, positive or challenging? Did it begin (although perhaps not immediately) after a relationship break-up or the passing of a loved one?

- Did it start after an episode of food poisoning or after a holiday where you had a very upset tummy?

- Do you worry about keeping everyone in your life happy? This sometimes leads you to not speak up for yourself as you would rather "swallow your words" and keep the peace.

My experience with the above scenarios follows.

Menstrual Cycle-related Bloat

If your tummy only bloats in the lead-up to your period, it is likely to be oestrogen dominance. Understand more about that and start there, based on the information in the "Hormone Havoc" section of this book.

After-meal Bloating

If bloating is an issue for you, in my experience working with clients I have learnt that some foods are better eaten on an empty stomach. Fruit is one of them. If bloating is a challenge for you, only eat fruit first thing in the morning on an empty stomach. None for lunch and none for afternoon tea. This includes dried fruit. You may find the same with starchy carbohydrates such as bread. Some people bloat no matter what time of day they eat bread, and, if that is the case, they will usually do well omitting all gluten-containing grains for a four-week period. Others are fine with bread or toast for breakfast, but for lunch it is a disaster on their digestive system.

All foods containing casein (ie, all foods from an udder — whether cow, goat or sheep, although the latter two tend to be tolerated better than cow's milk) can be significant contributors to a bloated stomach. Remove all sources from your diet for a trial period of four weeks, and observe how you feel. Coffee, too, can be incredibly bloating for some people. With a milk-based coffee, it may be the cow's milk or, less often, the soy milk, while even black coffee will cause some people to bloat. Biochemically, coffee drives both a liver and a gallbladder action, plus it asks the adrenals to secrete adrenalin, which can go on to affect another adrenal hormone, called aldosterone, which determines how much fluid your body retains. Switch to herbal tea or green tea, and give coffee a rest for four weeks. Green tea still has some caffeine in it (about one-third the caffeine of coffee), but the effects are buffered by another substance in the green tea called *theanine*. Green tea is also packed with antioxidants and contains what are believed to be powerful anti-cancer properties.

Observation is the key to this process, as your body does not have a voice. Your body communicates through symptoms, and lets you know when it is happy or not. A food that bloats you is, in that moment, not your friend, and your body is simply letting you know. Do not let your head run away with you when you notice this. Be reminded that just because it bloats you today does not mean you will never eat that food or drink that drink again. It simply means that right now, in this moment, it does not serve you. So take a four-week break from whatever you suspect. You will feel so different when you feed your body precisely what it wants. Never waste a bloated tummy. Ask it what it wants to tell you, as silly as that may sound. Your body has a wonderful wisdom.

Bloated Following a Stressful Experience

If your tummy has changed after a challenging time in your life, it is quite likely that your bloated abdomen was initially due to poor stomach acid production. Now, however, if poor stomach acid production has been ongoing because of an almost low-grade (or high-grade) anxiety inside you, the changes in digestion that were initially due to poor stomach acid production may have changed the gut bacteria and hence the pH of the large bowel. This scenario is one of the most common people share with me at my weekend events, and the situation that requires a multi-pronged approach.

Follow the tips in the "Foundation of Nourishment" section, in particular those about stimulating stomach acid. Read the sections about stress, and begin to work on your breath. Very importantly, but challenging at times, do your best to eat in a calm state, and you will also often see an improvement in symptoms if you follow the food recommendations from the after-meal bloating section above. If bloating began after a heartbreak, ask the discomfort what it wants you to know. You may feel a little odd having a conversation with your tummy, but your body knows the truth, and you might be surprised at the message it has for you.

Bloated Since Food Poisoning Episode or Upset Tummy While Travelling

Despite negative stool tests, I have seen this health picture frequently. Where once they had an iron gut, this person now feels like they react to everything. Even if you had forgotten that a gastroenteritis episode began your digestive system challenges, I suggest the following:

✿ Discuss with your GP having a *Helicobacter pylori* test.

✿ Take an herbal anti-parasitic tablet or liquid, even if your stool test has come back negative. Be guided by a health professional, but you usually need relatively high doses three times a day, and you need to take them for two months. If a parasite infection is the basis of your ongoing tummy trouble, the natural medicine must be taken for the full two months, as initially only the live parasites are killed by the herbs. As unpleasant as this is to think about, the parasites will have laid eggs in the lining of your bowel, and you want the herbs in your gut at the ready, in order to get rid of the parasites immediately as they hatch.

❉ Dietary change as outlined above can be very useful in this situation until the gut has healed. A gluten-free, casein-free, refined-sugar-free, and sometimes fruit-free trial period for four weeks can be highly beneficial. The Specific Carbohydrate Diet (SCD) has also been noted to have excellent results for gut health challenges, as does a low-FODMAP diet.

Bloating from "Swallowing Words"

Many women were raised to be good girls, to do as they are told, meet the needs of others and keep the peace. As a result, many live their adult lives in a rush, constantly trying to please everyone in their realm. If this describes you, you may notice that when you are interacting with another, and you don't agree with what is being said, you will at times swallow your words out of fear of an argument or "getting into trouble". Because this goes against your "gut" instinct, your tummy feels churned up, and metaphorically you have swallowed your words and they bloat your gut. Scientifically what has occurred is that you have likely produced adrenalin, which diverts the blood away from your gut to your periphery to help power you out of the danger your body now perceives it is in, and digestion of subsequent meals is compromised, leading to bloating.

If you find expressing yourself difficult, imagine that the words you want to say come from your heart, and move up to your throat and out of your mouth. Because they have come from your heart they have a beautiful intention behind them. Remember you cannot control how another person responds to what you say. That will be based on their life experiences, and the meanings they create from the words you say, based on their beliefs and their life experiences up until now. Swallowing your words harms your health, and it is not an authentic way to be in a relationship — friendship, with family, or an intimate relationship. I believe that one of the reasons we come together with another person is to learn and grow from and with each other. If you don't speak up, how does the other person grow and have the opportunity to

If you find expressing yourself difficult, imagine that the words you want to say come from your heart, and move up to your throat and out of your mouth.

see things from a different perspective? Plus, you will grow, too, as you further develop your courage.

Streptococcus

There is a bacterial species called *Streptococcus*. My experience in the lab, as well as working with people and their health, has taught me that no good comes from this bug.

Streptococcus causes tonsillitis and ear infections, and is often the basis of pneumonia and other respiratory infections. It lives in our sinuses and builds houses around itself, so that the immune system cannot destroy it effectively and we cannot evacuate it easily. It produces many toxins and lactic acid — more acid to add to the undesirable acid load. When we have a head full of mucous, especially when we are young, it can be difficult to cough up all of the sputum, and so we cannot help but swallow some. Our stomach acid is supposed to be highly acidic to sterilize anything bacterial that we swallow, yet the pH of the stomach acid is often too high to perform adequate sterilization. So the strep is able to move through the gut and take up residence wherever it likes. And there it lives, often forever, in our colon.

As well as being able to categorize gut bacteria into the groups *Firmicutes* and *Bacteroidetes*, we can classify them into those that love oxygen, known as *aerobes*, and those that don't use oxygen, called *anaerobes*. For good health, 70–90% of the aerobic flora in our large bowel needs to be *Escherichia coli*. It is believed that "reasonable" health can be obtained when there is 5% or less of the *Streptococcus* species. I have analyzed stool samples from countless people, adults and children, and I have seen aerobic flora counts of *Streptococcus* at 100% of the aerobic flora with zero *E. coli*, or, less extremely, I have seen strep counts of 70% and *E. coli* of 30%. Mostly due to my work with children with autism, I have seen first-hand that this bug is nasty. ASD behaviours are significantly less with less strep in the gut. In adults, strep makes them wet and mucousy mouth breathers, which pushes their blood chemistry to the acidic end of the spectrum, an aspect of biochemistry that also influences fat burning.

Of the bacterial phyla of *Firmicutes* and *Bacteroidetes* — remembering that *Firmicutes* are linked to fat storage and *Bacteroidetes* to leanness — strep falls into the *Firmicutes* division. So after all of these years of treating strep in the gut of my clients, knowing they would feel better, breathe better, and that their clothes would get looser, what I learnt while doing research for *Accidentally Overweight*, one of my earlier books, was that all along I have been significantly reducing the *Firmicutes* load in the gut of my clients with the dietary changes I suggest. Isn't the body amazing? Yet the calorie equation doesn't consider gut bacteria profiles in its calculation.

❖ Feed The Good Bugs In Short ... _____

Three to four kilograms of bacteria inhabit the large intestine. Science has shown that they can influence what calories are worth to the body. Taking care of your digestive system by eating real, whole foods that the body is capable of digesting is critical to optimal digestion, and therefore to the bacteria in the large intestine.

Gut bugs don't just play a direct role in what calories are worth to your body. They do this indirectly as well. Good gut bugs help support a healthy immune system; they support detoxification, particularly of heavy metals, which (to keep this simple) we are exposed to every day just through the number of cars on the road and/or via cigarette smoke, directly or passively. The bad gut bugs can disrupt the healthy lining of the gut, which can lead to increased gut permeability, hyper-stimulation of the immune system, which can lead to the excessive production of inflammatory substances, potential autoimmune diseases and add to the detoxification load rather than supporting it.

*P*lease remember that life is precious, that you are precious
and to treat yourself accordingly.

Dr Libby

Red Zone Green Zone

As you now understand, the calorie equation is a mathematical equation designed to calculate an individual's energy (ie, calorie) needs. It takes only a small number of factors into consideration, such as whether someone is healing from an injury or burns, as well as the amount of activity undertaken. It is astonishing, however, that among other things the *type* of exercise undertaken is not considered, given that, for example, interval training of short sprints utilizes fuel differently from running long distances, even if this training was done over the same duration. You will soon see some other essential factors the equation omits, yet it is still held as the gold standard for energy requirement calculations. My work suggests that the calorie equation is outdated.

In any given moment, your body is making a decision about which fuel to use to allow it to do its immediate work — keep your heart beating, lungs breathing, eyelids blinking, and brain thinking. It has two fuel options — glucose or fat — or a combination of both. What influences the choice your body makes? One of the biggest decision-makers in this is your nervous system. When it comes to your health, your ability to easily use body fat as a fuel, your degree of calm, and your quality of sleep, one body system stands out above all others: your nervous system.

What is the Nervous System?

The nervous system is comprised of various body parts, including your brain, your spinal cord, and the nerves that connect your brain to every organ of your body. There are several parts to your nervous system, which include the *central nervous system* (CNS) and the *autonomic nervous system* (ANS). The ANS has two branches, known as the *sympathetic nervous system* (SNS) and the *parasympathetic nervous system* (PNS). Rather than worrying about remembering all of these long-winded names, just know that the SNS drives the *fight-or-flight response*, which I also refer to as *living in the red zone*, while the PNS promotes the *rest, digest, repair and reproduce response*, also known as *living in the green zone*. This is diagrammatically represented in the following figure.

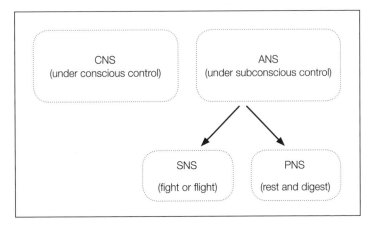

Different parts of the nervous system: The CNS and ANS are controlled differently, while the SNS and the PNS are branches of the ANS.

Your CNS is governed by your conscious mind; that is, you control it with your thoughts. For example, if you want to write, you choose to pick up a pen and write. If you choose to walk, you control the direction and the pace at which you travel. You choose it. Your ANS, however, is controlled by your subconscious mind. In other words you are *unable* to access it with your thoughts. You can't instruct it. Your ANS governs, for example, how quickly your heart beats, and how fast your hair and nails grow; rates over which you have no control. It heals a cut without you having to tell it to do so.

Too many people today live their lives constantly in the red zone, in a perpetual rush, trying to be all things to all people and meet the needs of everyone in their realm. I discussed this epidemic of "not enough-ness" in my TEDx talk. It is the ANS that is significantly affected by relentless haste, whether you reveal to the outside world that this is how you live, or keep it hidden behind a smile. We are enormously affected by the way our ANS responds to what we may not even realize we think about or perceive.

Let's look at the role the nervous system plays in the human body using fat as its fuel, particularly given that body fat that won't shift can be a source of frustration and stress for many people today, and can make them hurry around even more, and try to cram more in. When I share this information with audiences when I speak live, one of the joys in my life is witnessing their eyes light up with understanding and their hearts open to a whole new realm of possibility when it comes to their weight, their health, and how they feel and function every day — one that has zero to do with calories. People share with me that the extensive way the nervous system impacts on fat loss is one of the most powerful take outs from my weekend events, and information that leads to significant behaviour change.

The Nervous System and Body Fat

In any given moment the human body is making a decision about which fuel to use, based on the information it is receiving. Pause and consider that before we proceed. The hypothalamus in the centre of your brain asks the question, 24/7, "Am I safe?", and your *subconscious* has an answer for that. I don't necessarily mean physically safe, although this may be a factor for you if you have experienced stress through lack of physical safety in the past. You ask this question emotionally as well, and your subconscious has rules about what has to happen for you to feel safe. It may be about money, or owning your own home, or having your children with you, or about not being yelled at, for example. And the most powerful way to communicate to your body whether it is "safe" or not is via how you breathe. Remember I said you can't access your ANS with your thoughts? When you breathe in a short, shallow way, and the only part of you that moves is the top of your chest, adrenalin is driving that. That communicates to every cell in your body that your life is in danger. When you breathe diaphragmatically, when your abdomen expands when you inhale and shrinks back in when you exhale, you communicate to every cell in your body that you are safe, as you would never be able to breathe in this way if your life truly was in danger. So the way you breathe influences how your nervous system perceives your level of safety in that moment. Yet you might be making adrenalin, and hence breathing in a shallow way, simply because you have had a few coffees or because you have a few deadlines looming.

Think about running. Do you think when our ancestors woke in the morning, they thought, "Gosh, looks like a good day for a run"? Unlikely. They ran to escape danger or chase their food, and if you consider each of those scenarios, they are all over relatively quickly. Today, if you go for a run, your conscious mind knows you are doing so for fitness or to clear your mind, but the meaning your subconscious has most likely made is that your life is in danger. We are at a point in history where we are asking our body to create a new meaning from the information it obtains from the environment for the very first time in the entirety of human history. If you live a relatively calm existence and then you run, it will seem short-lived to your body. But if you live your life with intensity, feeling like there aren't enough hours in the day and that you can't keep up, and then you exercise with intensity as well, your body's perception will likely be that your attempt to escape from danger never ends. And when you live like this in the long term, it can lead to significant changes in your metabolism, as you will see explained in this book. For now, simply remember that your breath leads and your nervous system follows. In other words, the only way you can influence (ie, access) your ANS is via your breathing.

Remember, the only two fuels for the human body are glucose ("sugar") and fat. You don't use protein for fuel. The body breaks protein down into amino acids, which are then converted into glucose, so the body can use that glucose as fuel (energy). The body requires energy for everything it does, from walking to sleeping and from laughing to blinking; it all requires fuel.

A major health challenge today for too many people is that they spend too much time with the SNS activated, and the hormones behind that are the stress hormones adrenalin and cortisol. For the 150,000 years humans have been on the planet, adrenalin has communicated to every cell in the body that your life is in danger. It has prepared you to fight or flee. Today what leads us to make adrenalin is caffeine and the perception of pressure. You may be making adrenalin simply because you have to make a phone call that you would rather not make, or perhaps because you have gulped down three cups of coffee already today. The stress for most people in the Western world today is psychological rather than physical.

If the body's perception is that it needs to escape from impending danger, whether your thinking mind is telling you so or not, you need a fast-burning fuel available to do that. Your body thinks it has to get out of there and get out of there fast! So what fuel do you think your body

> *We* can burn fat effectively in a PNS-dominant state, because the body perceives it is safe when the PNS is activated.

will choose when it needs to flee, to get out of "danger" fast? Remember, its only choice is to burn either glucose or fat … In this scenario, it will choose glucose every time. The body thinks it has to in order to save your life, and we are all geared for survival. The body doesn't feel "safe" enough to use body fat as its fuel in this fight-or-flight state, because fat offers us a steady, slow release form of energy. We can burn fat effectively in a PNS-dominant state, because the body perceives it is safe when the PNS is activated. Yet, the PNS can never be the dominant arm of the ANS, it can never steer the ship, while the body perceives there may be a threat to your life, which is what adrenalin communicates, no matter what the reasons are behind you making it.

We have glucose stored in our muscles and liver in a form called *glycogen*, and these stores are mobilized whenever our body gets the message that it needs energy to fight or run, if there is not enough glucose to fuel our escape left in our blood from our last meal. This mobilization of glycogen out of the muscles due to stress can, over time, impact the function and appearance of our muscles, including allowing the onset of cellulite, particularly at the top of the legs. It can also be one of the mechanisms that leads someone to experience hypoglycaemia (low blood glucose), because, when the blood glucose starts to fall low, the liver is supposed to step in and release storage glycogen, and convert it back into glucose, to top up the blood. For a variety of reasons, chronic stress included, this mechanism can become inefficient. What you eat, of course, plays a significant role in hypoglycaemia as well, and dietary change coupled with stress management techniques, such as focusing on how you breathe, can often resolve the hypoglycaemia.

I believe that one of the most enormous health challenges of modern times is that the body can constantly be on the receiving end of the fight-or-flight message. There are so many factors, internal and external to us, that drive this response within us, and we will explore these in a moment. However, this means that we have to begin to actively choose to not go there, to not get caught up in the perceived urgency of tasks, and instead take steps in our daily lives to allow our nervous system to have some balance. When you have a balanced ANS, when you can easily swing between SNS dominance and PNS dominance, you effectively utilize both glucose and fat as fuels. And that is very healthy. It is when you are stuck in SNS dominance — with your body getting the message that it is therefore only safe to use glucose as a fuel — that health and weight challenges can arise that have nothing to do with calories.

Sympathetic Nervous System Dominance

Too many people today live in SNS dominance. Their perception of what they have to do in a day is overwhelming to them. They have usually also elevated their adrenalin production and pushed themselves further into SNS dominance with caffeine consumption during the morning. Even the most grounded, calm person will be fizzing, on the inside at least, with a few coffees under their belt. For some, even one caffeinated beverage is enough to amp them up so significantly that they overreact to the smallest thing, and both fat burning and calm are blocked.

For women, the calming, anti-anxiety sex hormone progesterone is typically low. This can be due to too much adrenalin and cortisol (explained in the "Hormone Havoc" section) and too much oestrogen (from food, the environment, and from compromised liver recycling with, as we saw in the "Detox Engine" section, the regular consumption of alcohol to "relax" at the end of the day); as a result, the "mad rush" feelings and the overreaction to things tend to be worse in the lead-up to menstruation. Throw in some sugary snacks, and perhaps more caffeine when the afternoon exhaustion kicks in, and you have a cocktail of behaviours aimed at reducing stress that are in fact adding a significant level of stress to the body.

On top of the physical stressors are the emotional responses that do not serve your health and keep you in a SNS-dominant state. As children these emotional patterns probably served a purpose of protection, but now as adults they are often detrimental to our mental and therefore our physical health, and often to our personal growth. I have listed, below, a few of the most common emotional patterns I observe in SNS-dominant women and in some men. It is important to point these out, because, if your emotional patterns and

The most powerful way to communicate to your body whether it is "safe" or not is via how you breathe.

beliefs are what
leads you to unknowingly communicate to your body that
it needs to burn glucose, which is what adrenalin does, the
best diet and movement regime won't get you the outcomes
you seek. The calorie equation cannot solve the metabolic
consequences of your belief that you are not enough. I want
you to understand where that belief has come from, and take
the steps to remove this cloud of false belief in which you live,
because you are completely and utterly enough.

Exhausting Emotional Patterns that Contribute to SNS Dominance

An inability to say "no"

I have heard it countless times from (mostly) female clients
and friends: "I don't know how to say 'no.'" There are many
times in our lives when we want to say "no" but instead we
say "yes", usually to please other people and to keep the peace.
We want others to like us, and we behave as though saying no
sometimes will either lead them to believe that we don't like
them or that they will think we are a terrible person. But when
we spell it out on paper like this, you can see how crazy it is!

A client shared with me a great example of this inability to
say "no". She was scheduled to go into the hospital to have a
baby and she had one day of solitude planned, the day before
she was to give birth. Her older children were going to be
at school, and she simply wanted a peaceful day at home by
herself to reflect and rest and be. So when her neighbour asked
if my client could look after her sick child for a few hours while
she went to a meeting, my client said "yes" … and begrudged
her neighbour for asking. Yet if she had simply explained to
her neighbour her plans for the day, it would have given her
neighbour an opportunity to explore other options.

It is time to stop giving up what you want to keep the peace.
Sure it is lovely to give. Contributing to the world and those
around you is a fundamental need for humans — contribution
helps give our lives meaning. Yet when we do it at our own
expense and say "yes" when secretly we wish we had said "no",

it doesn't serve anybody.

This pattern of not being able to say "no" is a major drain on our energy, not to mention our time. It revs our stress response, driving us into, or holding us in, SNS dominance. And our adrenal glands, which release the stress hormones, can also be significantly impacted upon over time. It is crucial to learn to say "no". However, knowing that this will help your health is usually not enough to promote change. You will tell yourself you need to say "no" far more often than you currently do, yet your subconscious drive to avoid pain (the perceived loss of love from those asking things of you) will usually lead you back to being a "yes" girl. Make it a mantra that if it's not a "hell, yes", then it's a "no".

Seeking acceptance, approval, appreciation and love

Another way the above words could be phrased is "seeking to avoid rejection" or "seeking to avoid being ostracized". When we constantly aim to prove our worth to the people in our lives or the people we meet, it is exhausting and adds another layer of stress to busy lives. However, when I am working with an individual, what I have noticed is that at first they usually can't reconcile their behaviour with wanting to fit in and be accepted. And then the penny drops — you can see it on their face — and the best way I can describe the expression is one of relief. And they look lighter, freer, somehow.

For the penny to drop, you often have to look down upon a situation in your own life as though you are an angel watching from above. Only when you look down upon yourself with a curious attitude, rather than with any form of judgement or preconceived ideas about what might be going on, will you see the situation as it really is — that you simply said or did what you did to be accepted, approved of, appreciated and ultimately loved. And there is nothing wrong with that. You just need to be aware of what drives you, so that if that behaviour also harms you in some way (for example, stresses you out and keeps you in SNS dominance), you have the power to change it. When you don't know why you do the things you do, when you just know that you always seem to end up doing things you don't want to do, or perhaps you feel used and unappreciated and unhappy, you are lost without a map. Looking down upon your precious self helps you see your path out.

Also explore whose love you craved the most when you were growing up. It is usually mum or dad. It doesn't mean you didn't have their love; just explore whose love you craved the most, and who you felt you had to be and what you had to do to be loved by that person. And what could you never do? Who could you never be? There is usually so much insight to be gained from this exploration, and it may help you see what drives some of your behaviours today.

Not putting you first

On an aeroplane the safety video always suggests that you put on your own oxygen mask first before helping others, the premise behind which is that if you pass out you will not be able to assist others. It is very easy to pay lip service to this concept; it is another story entirely to actually act on it. When you go to meditate or practise yoga or go to a café to read your favourite magazine, you are taking care of you and nurturing your soul, and this helps everyone around you. Typically, we are able to behave in a much calmer and kinder manner when we have put some runs on our own board and created a sense of spaciousness in our lives. When people tell me they have no time for this, of course I know they are busy. What I also know is that they have no space in their mind to fit in another task, another thing to remember. It is headspace people need, and only you can give yourself that. Start to incorporate relaxation rituals into your everyday life — don't wait until you actually feel stressed.

A girlfriend of mine had started to dread picking up her five children from school. With children aged between 9 and 17, she said, "Every day it was chaos, and the boys are at that age where they smell after school, and it was just so loud for the 20-minute drive home that I'd feel so stressed by the time we got there that I'd end up screaming at them on a daily basis. I couldn't cope, and yet I felt like such a dreadful mother for yelling at them. One day, to prepare myself for the school pickup, I listened to spa music while I drove, and it was still on when the older children got into the car. After initially teasing me about my taste in music and making a few *om* noises, we had the calmest drive home we'd had since they hit puberty. So now that is part of my daily ritual. It doesn't always completely negate the chaos, but it is certainly much less, and I, too, am different. I'm not drowning now. I respond to them differently, from a much more centred space."

Guilt

Guilt is such a futile emotion. What leads you to feel guilty? Most often it is your perception that you have let someone else down. Yet when you pause to think about that, it is simply a story you have made up. The reality is that it is not physically possible to let another human being down. If you do or say something, it is the other person's choice *entirely* whether they feel disappointment or any other emotion. And their response is 100% based on their conditioning, and their life experiences up until now, just as yours is. You have never walked in anyone else's shoes, nor have they walked in yours. You have no idea what it is like to be them, or what emotional patterns they run and why. If they choose disappointment, well, they choose disappointment. It is just an emotion and it will pass, and if they feel disappointed about something you have or have not done, it is usually because they feel disappointed with themselves. Disappointment will be an emotion they feel regularly, and that is not your responsibility.

Many adults feel guilty because they believe they are not a good enough friend, partner, spouse, parent, daughter, son, sister, brother, colleague ... And it gets you nowhere. The first step to change your exhausting emotional responses, the ones that don't serve you, is awareness. And although you may still throw to guilt, you can catch yourself.

> The first step to change your exhausting emotional responses, the ones that don't serve you, is awareness.

You can recognize much sooner that you have responded to a situation
with guilt, and, rather than letting it linger and permeate your life, your relationships and your self-esteem, you can realize you have simply told yourself your old story. Make this one of your mental go-to statements: Only if I were to consistently indulge in the debilitating, exhausting, health-depleting emotion of guilt will I feel it, instead of remembering that I haven't walked in anyone else's shoes, cannot control how they will respond to my words or actions, and that only I determine how *I* feel.

From this point on, begin to become aware of the stories you tell yourself. They are simply that: stories. And remember you have zero control over how someone reacts to what you do or say. Guilt is exhausting. Become aware of how often you feel it. Notice if guilt motivates you or makes you want to stay at home and eat. Or if you attempt to distract yourself from the guilt you feel through your nightly few glasses of wine. Start to notice …

How Does SNS Dominance Unfold?

Most people today need to spend far more time with their PNS activated. How can we do this? For a start, we need to identify the numerous roads to an SNS-dominant life, and then address those that feature in our own lives. While some of them involve a high or low level of a particular physical substance, such as caffeine or progesterone, others are the result of our emotional landscape and the behaviours we display, which are the result of our beliefs. Trouble is, most of us are totally unaware of what we really believe. My book *Rushing Woman's Syndrome* offers insights and assistance for women on the emotional side of things, while below is a summary of the physical aspects of our lifestyles that can lead to SNS dominance.

Caffeine

I wish it weren't so, believe me! But yes, caffeine is the fastest and surest way to amp up that SNS response. And how many people start their day with a caffeinated beverage? More than 90% of people in the Western world consume caffeine every day. It is a powerful nervous-system drug, and it also drives the adrenal glands to produce adrenalin, the hormone that promotes the SNS to stay in the red-alert alarm state. Caffeine demands that your body use glucose as its fuel, drawing on glucose in the blood or drawing the stored version of glucose (glycogen) out of the liver and the muscles into the blood to be used as the fuel in this highly alert state.

What I have observed in so many women, in particular, is that if their day is calm, non-chaotic and without pressure or demands, and then caffeine is thrown into the mix, the caffeine still stimulates (as that is its mechanism of action), but not to the point of overwhelming, which can show up as snappy, impatient behaviour or sadness and withdrawal. But how do you know when a day may present with no challenges and therefore might be "safer" to have a caffeinated drink? One client, Melissa, described it beautifully ...

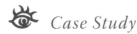 *Case Study*

Jo's Story

I like to start my day with a latte that I make myself. I sometimes then buy a coffee mid-morning when I am out and about. If I don't speak to anyone all day, I feel OK. I do notice my energy crashes about two hours after the second coffee, but so far as the feelings of being overwhelmed go, they don't kick in. But these days, at the age of 41, I only have to get a phone call from my husband, and, if he is panicked about something or seems frustrated with me, I can't stop shaking on the inside after I hang up. I feel like the smallest task on my to-do list is overwhelming, and I make mountains out of molehills for the rest of the day. I can end up in tears feeling like I can't cope even though I felt fine when I woke up.

When I came to see you about my periods, you asked me to take a break from coffee for two menstrual cycles. Not only did my premenstrual tension go away, but those feelings, even when my husband was worked up, did not arise the whole time I was off coffee. I can't tell you the difference it has made to my day and to my health. I now have one coffee on the weekend if my husband and I take the children out for breakfast, but it took that break for me to realize that the coffee was like the straw that broke this camel's back!

Step one to down-regulate your SNS is to take a break from coffee, and at first switch to green tea. It does contain caffeine (about 30 milligrams per cup), but much less than coffee (about 80 milligrams in an espresso-based drink with one shot of coffee; and keep in mind that many cafés give you two shots of coffee as standard practice). Plus green tea is rich in antioxidants, has significant anti-cancer properties, and benefits the liver. Some people find that even green tea is too stimulating, so once you have weaned off coffee using green tea, you can switch to herbal teas that contain no caffeine, if you prefer to. Or simply make warm water with lemon as your hot drink. You can go cold-turkey off coffee if that is your style, too, of course. Some people — not all, though — experience headaches when they do this. You can either decide to ride it out, drink a lot of water, or a magnesium supplement can also bring relief. If that is what coming off coffee does to you, it is worth considering what drinking it was doing to you.

Not everyone needs to stop all caffeine and stay off it. I suggest giving up caffeine initially so you can see if you feel different. Countless clients have told me that, while they had thought they had anxiety and insomnia, once they stopped having coffee there was no trace of either.

Low Progesterone for Women

When a woman's sex hormones are out of balance, it can feel to her like the world will end. She can feel "out of her body", as though she has no grounding, and like there is something wrong but she doesn't know what it is. Progesterone clearly has a reproductive role to play in our body; however, it plays many other roles as well. It behaves like an antidepressant and an anti-anxiety agent, and it is crucial for clear thinking. It is also a diuretic, meaning it helps you get rid of excess fluid. In the 16 years I have worked with people one-on-one about their health and nutrition, I have seen six women with optimal progesterone levels. Six! In 16 years! I know I see a biased group of the population: no one comes to see a health professional like me when they feel fabulous and everything in their world is perfect.

Nonetheless, it has become common but not normal for a woman's progesterone to be low, and that can mean any or all of the following: low mood, unexplained weight gain, an inability to lose weight despite excellent food and movement patterns, challenges conceiving, fluid retention, poor thyroid function, or an anxious feeling inside her body that she can't explain. And if she stops to think about it, she can't work out whether the feeling like she never gets it all done and can never quite manage to keep everyone happy — whether that anxious feeling — came first or if something is causing it. And from a scientific perspective, it can be either. It can certainly be that all of the perceived urgency brought on the anxious feeling, as year after year living our life in this way is a sure-fire way to deplete our progesterone levels. However, low progesterone levels can also lead us to feel anxious, as progesterone physiologically helps to keep women calm. It is a classic chicken-or-egg situation. More about this in the "Hormone Havoc" section.

Lack of Sleep

There are a few things I link to amazing health: optimal nutrition (of course), fresh air, movement, love, forgiveness, and great sleep. Sleep affects our physical and mental health, and countless research studies have shown that a lack of sleep can lead to weight gain. The calorie equation doesn't factor in what a lack of sleep does to metabolism.

The links between good-quality sleep and stress management are also abundant. Sleep is often the only time our bodies are able to access the rest and repair part of our nervous system (the PNS). Sleep is critical for skin regeneration, immunity, fertility, hair growth, nail growth, and all other non-vital processes the body will not prioritize during the day, if under constant stress and SNS activation. For many of us, when we put our head on the pillow at night it may be the first time that day we feel we have truly stopped. Yet the more tasks that pile up on our to-do list, the more we tend to sacrifice the one thing that allows our PNS to become dominant again: sleep. It is important to learn how to "relax in the doing".

However, even at bedtime PNS activation doesn't occur for everyone. When I was researching sleep to create a sleep webinar for my website based on statistics in New Zealand, I learnt that in 2012 in a country of about 4.5 million people, not all of whom are adults (obviously), 680,000 prescriptions were written out for sleeping tablets. There are multiple reasons for this, and one of them is SNS dominance.

When I would run programmes at health retreats, I would often ask people what they loved most about their week. One of the most common answers I received was "sleep". Going to bed at a good time and getting up at the same time each morning, usually with the sun, sends a powerful message to your endocrine system, the system that involves all of the glands that regulate hormones and the incredibly important body systems involved in reproduction, and the stress response. When you don't sleep enough, you don't allow your PNS to have as much of a chance to be the dominant arm of the nervous system. So for people who live their lives with urgency, the time they are asleep may be the only time they give their PNS the opportunity to drive the ship.

Yet for many SNS-dominant people, they can't sleep properly or they do not feel that sleep restores them. Remember that when you are in an SNS-dominant state your body tends to churn out stress hormones, and if one of those stress hormones is screaming to every cell of your body that your life is in danger, which is what adrenalin does, your body will never let you sleep deeply because it wants you to survive the imminent attack it perceives. So it is a vicious cycle. Sleep is difficult to restore to be of excellent quality if you don't first allow the PNS to become the dominant arm of the nervous system. Re-establishing restorative sleep provides countless health benefits, and many find weight loss — unrelated to their calorie intake — is one of them.

Over-exercising

As mentioned earlier, certain types of exercise can seem like more stress to an already over-stressed human body. For all of human history, running meant we were attempting to escape from danger, while now it has become a way to burn off the excesses a Western lifestyle "affords" us.

I am not saying running is bad, for those of you who love it, although I don't think most runners are aware of the biochemical changes running drives, such as free radical and inflammatory mediator generation. However, there is certainly a science that can be applied to running to promote fat burning and nervous system calm, and barefoot running certainly promotes being present in the moment. Plus it is the body's response to the training that needs to be observed.

I am simply saying that if running and high-intensity exercise, combined with good eating, hasn't shifted your weight by now, it is not suddenly going to start doing so until some other work on your body's chemistry and nervous system is done. The calorie equation won't hold true if there are metabolic factors that confound it. And in addressing the aspects of metabolism that you need to, you get healthy, which is what then allows your body to shed the weight. Weight loss is the consequence of being healthy.

Even though your conscious mind knows you are simply exercising intensely, from your body's perspective the release of stress hormones with exercise indicates the presence of a threat which needs to be dealt with. Once this is done, the PNS slows our heart rate and respiration back down, brings the blood back to the digestive tract so that we can digest our food, works to repair any tissue damage, and increases libido. Night-time is when the PNS is supposed to have the time to do its job, but this relies on us going to bed early enough as well as our perception of pressure and urgency. As you read earlier, the sympathetic and parasympathetic systems are supposed to balance each other, and in those people who have a balanced nervous system, high-intensity exercise will lead to fat loss, as the parasympathetic rest time between workouts is when muscle tissue is built. However, there are other, potentially less damaging ways to boost metabolism and decrease body fat, summarised in later pages.

Those who are unable to lose fat by doing regular high-intensity exercise may have a dominant SNS, and consequently an inhibited PNS. There is too much systemic stress coming from somewhere, and for those people adding high-intensity exercise is counterproductive, as it adds to their sympathetic load, pushing them even more out of balance. Instead you want to decrease the sympathetic load by reducing stressors and choosing exercise that includes those done slowly and that involve controlled breathing, such as restorative yoga, qigong, t'ai chi, Kundalini yoga, Feldenkrais, or Alexander technique. These activities will increase the parasympathetic system and help balance the ANS. The goal is to balance the nervous system so that when you do need to rush, when things truly are urgent, you can attend to them, but then leave the rush, and all its health-depleting effects, behind, rather than living every day with a perceived urgency.

Start to explore your perception of pressure. Not that long ago, people linked stress and pressure to situations where, for example, they might be ill or a loved one is sick. Now when I ask people where the stress and pressure is in their life, many people reply "emails". You care about emails because you are a caring human and you want to be efficient and get back to people and not let anyone down. They make you busy, but they are rarely pressure. Consider the difference in language and the impact on your nervous system of "I am busy" versus "I am under pressure" — worlds apart. I am not saying there isn't real pressure in this world. Of course there is. Just save your perception of it for when you really need it. Don't put your nervous system through the stress of feeling pressure daily from a busy, opportunity-filled life, rich with incredible experiences.

Lack of Solitude

Another factor that can lead to SNS dominance is a lack of solitude, time spent on your own. When I talk about being alone I don't mean feeling lonely. They are different things. In fact, science has demonstrated some of the health benefits that come from spending time in solitude. It decreases stress hormones and has been shown to boost memory, creativity, mood and empathy. It allows us to recharge. On the inside this means that the PNS gets to have its time in the sun being dominant, where the vital rest, repair and digest processes can do their work. When we rest and repair, the body is able to choose between using sugar or fat as its fuel, and it usually chooses both. That is a good thing. Health problems can occur when the body feels as though it has no choice but to predominantly choose glucose for its fuel. It is not only that your clothes become tighter when you don't use fat as a fuel. The by-products of glucose metabolism include lactic acid and other substances linked to inflammation and oxidation, the processes through which we age from the inside out. You want your body to be able to burn both fuels efficiently.

How can you seek solitude in your day? Going for a walk by yourself and noticing the Nature around you is a great place to start. If you live with other people and you have the house to yourself, even if it is only once a week for a brief period of time, allow yourself to stop for at least some of that time, even though you might feel like "making the most of it to get more jobs done". You may feel that I cannot possibly understand your life and how busy you are. But part of what I want to show you is that when you create a spaciousness in your life, you *feel* as though you have more time, and you no longer feel that everything is so urgent.

It may not feel possible for you right now, particularly if you have small children. Often when they rest you need to rest, too, although so many people rush around even more while their baby sleeps, to get on top of the jobs that have piled up! One way to approach this might be to give yourself permission to rest on two out of the seven days of the week, while your baby sleeps. For the other five, you can choose to do tasks or to rest. Or you may prefer to start with one day of rest and increase this by one day every second week, until you have three rest days a week, as small steps can feel much more manageable. Another important thing to consider is that children are little for such a relatively short time. If you feel like right now you just can't take some time in solitude, you will soon be able to. If you feel like this, then perhaps while they sleep you can at least sit for five minutes and focus on your breathing. More begets more, remember? It can be practical to start small with your solitude if you feel as though it is a far-off dream.

Excess Liver-loaders

Optimal liver function is vital to fat burning. "Stress" on the physical body can also play a role in pushing us into SNS dominance through a variety of scientific mechanisms, the details of which I have explained in my book *Accidentally Overweight*. Rather than focusing on the mechanisms here, I simply want you to know that some foods and certain beverages can promote a stress response inside us. For example, you may notice that your heart races after you have had too much wine in one sitting for your body to detoxify. Countless women tell me that they notice their heart racing once they go to bed after they have had alcohol. The main liver-loaders are listed below and are discussed in more detail in the "Detox Engine" section. They include:

* alcohol
* caffeine
* trans fats
* refined sugars
* synthetic substances, such as pesticides, medications, skin-care products
* infection: for example, viruses such as glandular fever (also known as Epstein–Barr virus and mononucleosis).

Some of these you have a choice about, some not so. When it comes to the amount of alcohol, caffeine and refined sugars in your diet, you know when you are having too much — and I mean too much for you. The amount tolerated by one person is likely to be different from another, and you know better than anyone when you are having too much of anything. Even as you read this, if something has welled up inside you, your body's wisdom is letting you know. Of course knowledge is one thing; action is another thing entirely. Taking action to lower or omit your liver-loaders for a period of time can make a significant difference to living in SNS dominance and its health consequences.

Women and Alcohol

The regular over-consumption of alcohol is too common for too many women today. Many are exhausted, overwhelmed, and haven't had any time to themselves for at least 5 or 25 years, and alcohol is (to paraphrase many of my clients) "my only pleasure in the day", "the only way I can relax at the end of the day", "something for me ... the only thing just for me in my day", "the only way I get any peace" or "reward for all of my efforts over the day". When I ask women who drink every night to finish the sentence "Alcohol is ...", those are some of the things they say. The reality is alcohol is none of those things. They are meanings *you* have given alcohol. These are the stories you tell yourself about why you need it and why it is OK to have it every night of your life.

I don't believe the female body, in particular, was ever designed to consume alcohol most nights of its adult life. And women are experiencing the consequences of the regular over-consumption of it, with this type of drinking now highly associated with five of our biggest cancers. The links are undeniable. But for many, even scientific fact that the regular over-consumption of alcohol (amounts outlined in the "Detox Engine" section) significantly increases the risk of breast cancer won't stop you from telling yourself that it is your "only pleasure in the day". Ladies, seriously. If the only thing you derive pleasure from in your entire day is an alcoholic drink, it is time for a new perspective. (As an aside, many women repeat the same statements to me about coffee or a particular type of food.) This is not about taking away your fun or your pleasure. It is not about going without. I simply want you to be able to choose how much and how often you consume these liver-loaders, rather than your desire for them being ruled by your emotional state — for then you feel out of control, and often regret your food or drink choices, and judge yourself harshly as a result. This creates even more stress and holds you deeper into SNS dominance, further blocking the utilization of body fat as a fuel.

Choice

We have so much to be thankful for. I encourage you to be truly thankful *every* day for the privilege of living in a peaceful country, of having your basic needs met. Every night before you go to sleep, take a moment to simply be grateful for what you *do* have and not worry about what you may not have. Take some time out *every* day to have an "attitude of gratitude". We are so blessed to live in a society where we have an amazing array of choices available each day — more than our ancestors would ever have dreamed possible. And it is likely that anyone reading this, no matter how they may perceive their own life at present, still has a lifestyle that millions in the world would wish could be theirs. Many people don't even have clean water to drink.

> *E*very night before you go to sleep, take a moment to simply be grateful for what you *do* have and not worry about what you may not have.

It is also easy to take choice for granted, particularly when life doesn't work out quite the way we had planned. We have opportunities to shape our futures, but we don't always have control over unexpected events. We would never consciously choose for ourselves or those we love to have an accident, a serious illness, lose their job, or be involved in a natural disaster. But even if challenges present themselves, we must never forget that we retain control over our attitude toward that event. When I talk with people about their perception of choice, I am fascinated, occasionally saddened, but mostly inspired by the immense power of the human spirit. Here is one such response ...

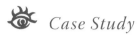 *Case Study*

Hannah's Story

When my parents died when I was 16, I had no choice in the circumstance. However, I was faced with other choices: to seek the so-called comfort of drugs or the true support of friends, to be negative or positive, to look backward or forward. Although I had absolutely no choice surrounding the situation I found myself in, I still had a choice in terms of what attitude I adopted. I knew that whatever choice I made wouldn't bring them back, so I simply chose to get on with my own life as best I could. Admittedly, there were times when I doubted I would succeed in doing so, but there is no comparison between that which is lost by not succeeding and that which is lost by not trying. With no family to fall back on, or blame, I learnt earlier than most that I was totally responsible for my own choices for the rest of my life. Because of the volunteer work I have ended up doing in the later part of my life, I have walked the beat with police as rocks were hurled at us, intervened in domestic violence situations, and sat for hours on a drug bust. Perpetrators of those crimes made different choices than me, but I suspend judgment because I may have made the same choices once, and I give thanks that I didn't. Choices have given me more than my fair share of joy and sorrow. But even in my darkest moments, I remind myself to give thanks for that freedom to choose.

Every day, I am truly grateful for so much in my life, such as fresh air, freedom, and real food. I am equally grateful for the things I don't have, like persecution, hunger and disease. Every day, it is worth reminding ourselves that the choices are ours. I cannot encourage you enough to spend time each day focusing on the things for which you are grateful. Share that gratitude with others. And remember to include the things that aren't in your life for which you are grateful, too. As Tony Robbins so accurately says, "what you focus on is what you feel". And if you tell yourself that alcohol is the only pleasurable thing in your entire day, then it will be, yet there is so much more on offer, around you and within you every minute of every day and night. It is just that when you are exhausted and running on the caffeine, sugar, alcohol highway of sub-optimal nutrition and SNS dominance, racing around everywhere with your to-do list never being all checked off, it can be quite a challenge to remember how magnificent your life truly is.

Allow your PNS to be dominant, whether that is through consuming less caffeine, sorting out your sex hormone balance, going to bed earlier, or scheduling some breath-focused move-ment in your day. Exploring and resolving elements of your emotional landscape are also going to assist. And from the spaciousness that PNS dominance promotes, you can not only see the magnificence and the wonder, but you can feel it within, just as you did as a young child. Your rituals create your life. Get some good ones!

Life a Long Time Ago and Life Today

There is an age-old inclination wired into us to protect, hoard and defend. The enemy is lurking, waiting to eat you, to annihilate you. The part of our brain linked to the fight-or-flight response, known as the *reptilian brain*, is — despite being augmented by the limbic brain (a different part of the brain linked to emotions) and the neocortex (yet another part of our very clever brain) — still focused on physical survival, the fight or flight. And when we allow our most basic impulses, the very ones that helped the earliest humans survive, to direct the higher brain centres, we act like lizards. And given we were born with the inclination to do whatever is needed to survive, we need to respect the genius of a brain that has done its job and brought us this far.

But we also need to update our wiring since the chances of being eaten by a lion are slim, even though when we live with urgency our body's perception is that that big cat is actually very real indeed. Being on red alert has now become maladaptive, because it causes us to live in a constant state of tension, which is unhealthy and therefore counterproductive to our survival. However, our nervous system, of which our brain is a part, hasn't been able to keep up with the rate of change or the pace of life that the Western world now asks of us. So for now, until our evolution can "catch up", we have to choose to support the part of our nervous system that dissolves tension as long as we feel it is safe to do so. This is key to amazing health, and is critical for many people to be able to lose weight.

There is a wonderful analogy I love to use to describe how people have become oblivious to the stress in their lives. It is about a frog and, as green tree frogs are one of my favourite creatures on the planet, it appeals to me even more. The analogy, whose origin is unknown, is this. If you put a frog in cool water, it swims around very happily. If you put a frog in boiling water, it immediately jumps out to save itself. But if you put a frog in cool water and slowly bring that water to the boil, the frog doesn't notice and doesn't jump out. I believe that most people in the Western world would jump out of the pressure in their lives if they were suddenly thrown into it. But we don't jump out when it gradually increases over the years. We don't tend to notice until a crisis hits — the death of someone we love or when our own health crashes, for example. Don't let it take a health crisis to wake you up to the fact that without your health you have nothing.

If you recognize that you are like a frog whose world has been on the boil, act now to change it. Begin to put strategies in place to change either your situation or your perception of your life, or both. Either way, the changes it will foster in your biochemistry, your body's ability to use fat as a fuel, your emotional landscape, and hence your health, are potentially very powerful.

❖ Red Zone Green Zone In Short ... ____

The nervous system plays a highly significant role in the choice your body makes about which fuel to use. It can only choose glucose or fat, or a combination of both.

When you are in SNS dominance — the *fight-or-flight response*, or the red zone — your body gets the message via adrenalin that your life is in danger, and it needs to power you to get out of there. So your body supplies you with a fast-burning fuel to do this. Your fast-burning fuel is glucose. When you live your life with too many hours in SNS (*sympathetic nervous system*) dominance, your body has no choice but to mostly use glucose as its fuel, not fat, as fat is a slower-burning fuel. Think of glucose as petrol on the flames of a fire, whereas fat is akin to wood being the fuel for a fire.

What leads us into SNS dominance? Caffeine and our perception of pressure. Get honest about how much caffeine you are consuming, and notice how it affects you. Take a break from caffeine to get a clear picture of this. Explore your perception of pressure. Where do you perceive it? Is it really pressure, or do you make it pressure because you care so much? Save pressure for real stress and pressure, not emails and general busy-ness.

What activates the PNS, the *rest, digest, repair and reproduce* arm of the nervous system? Diaphragmatic breathing. Remember you can't access the autonomic nervous system (ANS) with your thoughts. You can't tell it what to do. You can't tell the ANS that, even though you are churning out adrenalin because you have had a few coffees this morning and a few new deadlines hit your plate within the hour, you are safe and it's just work. It doesn't work like that.

When you have high circulating levels of adrenalin, your body believes your life is in danger, and you breathe with short, shallow breaths. When you breathe diaphragmatically, you communicate to every cell in your body that you are safe, as you would never be able to breathe that way — you would never think to do so — if your life truly was threatened. The way you breathe is your only road into the ANS. It is the only way you can influence the perception of the ANS about whether you are safe or not, and your body won't feel safe enough to burn body fat if the SNS is activated.

To activate the PNS, you need to move your diaphragm when you breathe. Many people need to schedule this to get back into the habit of breathing in this way across the day. It is not about breathing this way just when you go to yoga, and then as soon as that is done it is back to adrenalin-driven shallow breaths. A new level of health comes when we live from PNS dominance and allow the SNS to be activated for short periods, returning to PNS activation as our predominant way of life.

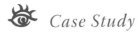 *Case Study*

Mrs C's Story

Mrs C came to see me after she had done a marathon. She had not done the marathon for weight loss: it had been on her bucket list, and she felt a great sense of achievement that she had done it. Mrs C had trained for nine months in the lead-up to the marathon, and had run between 64 kilometres and 145 kilometres per week, every week, for those nine months.

When she came to see me after she had completed the marathon, she showed me the diary she kept of her food consumption during this time, and it was clear that she was burning far more fuel than she was consuming. Yet, over the nine months of training, she had gained 12 kilograms.

Diagnosis
There were potentially numerous factors at play for Mrs C, but one was certainly that she was living in SNS dominance,

driving her body to use predominantly glucose as a fuel and not access her body fat to burn, as her body perceived it was not safe enough to do so. The way she was training had just added to her body's perception.

It is not the exercise itself that is the problem, but the body's response to the training. Running in this way dramatically increases free radical production, which are the by-products of energy production and are destructive on a cellular level. They cause damage to cell membranes, and hence to all tissues. During prolonged exercise, some studies suggest that 5–10% of energy production is derived from muscles being broken down, leading to a loss of lean muscle mass, which slows the metabolic rate. There can also be excessive wearing of the joints, which can cause inflammation, leading to an increase in cortisol production, as it acts as an anti-inflammatory. But cortiosl is also catabolic, further wasting muscle tissues, decreasing metabolic rate further, and driving fat storage.

Course of action
For Mrs C, I didn't need to change her food. She ate very well. Instead, I suggested she do resistance training to increase her muscle mass, yoga and/or Pilates for flexibility, breathing exercises so she could retrain herself to diaphragmatically breathe again, and walk in Nature. I also increased her anti-oxidant and essential fatty acid intake. She stopped weighing herself, too.

Outcome
A year after she had done her marathon, out of curiosity Mrs C decided to weigh herself. And she wrote to me to tell me that she was 15 kilograms lighter than when she had run the marathon.

Pay attention to how *your* body responds to the training you do.

If you are troubled by external circumstances, it is not the circumstances that trouble you, but your own perception of them — and they are in your power to change at any time.

Marcus Aurelius

Can Stress Increase Body Fat?

The production of stress hormones can significantly influence whether your body gets the message that it needs to store body fat or burn it. You make stress hormones from your adrenal glands, which are two walnut-sized glands that sit on top of your kidneys. The two main stress hormones the body makes are adrenalin and cortisol. They behave very differently from one another, and communicate very different messages, but both have the power to influence whether your clothes get tighter or looser, even if the way you eat and move has not changed. They influence your metabolism beyond the considerations of the calorie equation, yet they must be factored in in today's world where so many people describe experiencing stress daily.

A US study published by the American Psychological Association in 2011, conducted with 1226 people over the age of 18 years, found that the top five areas of stress (in descending order) were money, work, the economy, relationships (spouse, children, girl-/boyfriend) and family responsibilities.

In 2013, in a study conducted by the Australian Psychological Society, involving 21,000 people aged over 18 years of age who were working, Australians reported significantly lower levels of well-being and significantly higher levels of stress and distress than in 2012 and 2011. Almost three-quarters of Australians (73%) reported that stress was having at least some impact, with almost one in five people (17%) reporting that stress was having a strong to very strong impact on their physical health. Finances were the leading cause of stress for Australians, followed by family and health issues. I share these results with you to demonstrate how significantly stress has permeated our existence in the Western world, and, given it has such major metabolic and health consequences, these mechanisms need to be understood so people can be far more accurately guided with their health choices to obtain the outcomes they seek. Addressing stress hormone production can be a critical factor in modern-day weight loss. Of course we can argue that there has always been stress, but it has never before come in the constant, urgent avalanche that has become the norm for so many people in the Western world.

Stress hormones don't just impact metabolism directly. They can also interfere with other processes in the body that are vital to your metabolic rate, such as thyroid function, gut function, and sex hormone balance. These body systems can also influence whether we feel calm or anxious, happy or sad, and these emotional states can also impact food choices and our level of self-care and self-esteem.

The Three Parts of the Brain

Central to our response to stress is what is known as the *fight-or-flight response*: when faced with a perceived threat to our safety, we either stand our ground and meet the threat head-on, or we flee to safety. Our body's — and in particular our hormones' — response to perceived stress is influenced by the three integrated parts of the human brain, so we will briefly look at these before moving on to the stress hormones themselves.

The first part is the *brain stem*, or *reptile brain*. This is the *survival brain*. It controls the functions responsible for our survival, as an individual and as a species — things such as hunger, thirst, heartbeat, breathing, digestion, immunity and sex drive. It is the basic, primal part of us that is in all animals: give me food, give me shelter, let me reproduce. This part of the brain also *initiates* the fight-or-flight stress response.

The second part is the *limbic system*, or *mammalian brain*. All mammals have it, and it is composed of the amygdala, the hippocampus and the thalamus. This is our *emotional brain*. It controls all of the functions related to emotional aspects of survival, such as memory, behaviour, pleasure and pain responses, and our experience of all emotions. It *maintains* the fight-or-flight stress response.

The third part is the *cerebral cortex*, or *human brain*. Humans and some other mammals, such as apes, dolphins and whales, have this brain, and it is our *thinking brain*. It controls such things as decision-making, attention, awareness, language, judgment, reading and writing. It is the centre of higher thought, and it is *impaired* by the fight-or-flight stress response.

These comprise the mental processes that feed into our physiological response to life. Now we will explore these physiological mechanisms in more detail, but later we will return to the mental and physical partnership when we look at coping mechanisms, as these, too, impact on whether your body gets the message to burn fat or store it.

The Adrenal Glands

Let's look at what we ask of our body from an adrenal and stress hormone perspective when we live a high-stress, fast-paced lifestyle, or if we live life on an emotional roller-coaster. For those of you who have read *Accidentally Overweight, Rushing Woman's Syndrome* or *Beauty from the Inside Out,* some of this information was covered there, but this section has been expanded and is essential reading at this stage in your journey to understanding the way stress hormones can have an impact on your body shape and size.

As you now know, your adrenal glands are two walnut-sized glands that sit just on top of your kidneys. They may be small, but the power they pack when they are working optimally is an energetic, vitality-inducing, health gift to us all. The adrenal glands produce many hormones, two of which are your stress hormones, namely adrenalin and cortisol.

Adrenalin, Sugar Cravings and Blood Glucose

As you leant in the "Red Zone Green Zone" section, adrenalin is your short-term, acute stress hormone. It is the one that is produced when you get a fright. If someone suddenly runs into the room and startles you, the feeling that follows is caused by adrenalin. Adrenalin is designed to get you out of danger — and get you out of danger fast. Historically, humans made adrenalin when their lives were threatened. The response, fuelled by adrenalin, was typically physical. If a tiger suddenly jumped out at you in the jungle, or perhaps a member of another tribe started chasing you with a spear, the body made adrenalin, promoting the fight-or-flight response.

When activated, the typically excellent blood supply to your digestive system is diverted away from your digestive system to your periphery, to your arms and your legs. This is necessary because you need a powerful blood supply to your arms and legs to get you out of danger. Hence digestion is compromised.

You also need fuel to help you escape, and the most readily available, fastest-burning fuel inside the body is *glucose*, often referred to as sugar, a carbohydrate. Your liver and muscles store glucose in the form of *glycogen*, and adrenalin communicates to your liver and muscles when energy is required. Glycogen is converted back into glucose, and this glucose is released back into your blood. Your blood glucose (ie, sugar) subsequently shoots up, ready to fuel your self-defence or your escape. And you feel amped up, although many people today don't identify this, as they have become accustomed to it being their norm.

This cascade of events — and the biochemical changes that result — allows you to escape from danger in a very active way. Regardless of the outcome, regardless of whether you win that challenge or not (you escape, die, or win the fight), this stress, the threat to your life and the need for adrenalin is over quickly. The trouble is that, for many of us in the modern world, it is more often psychological stress that drives us to make adrenalin, and for many people today that stress is never switched off. Although our life may not literally be threatened, this hormone still communicates to every cell of our body that our life is indeed at risk. Adrenalin makes your heart race, your thoughts race, and gives you a jittery feeling that can make it difficult to feel calm and centred, despite your best efforts.

Psychological stress can come in many forms. It may be that you return from a week away from work to find 700 new emails in your in-box, and you wonder when on Earth you are going to find the time to deal with those. It may be that your landline rings, and while you take that call your mobile rings, and you feel that you can barely finish one conversation before demands come in to start another one. If you are sitting in front of your computer while all of this is going on, and a few emails arrive in your in-box while you juggle the incoming demands and noise, adrenalin tends to climb higher. Or perhaps you set your alarm for the morning, you press the snooze button ... you keep pressing snooze ... and suddenly you sit bolt upright in bed and realize you are running late. Maybe you still have clothes to iron, lunches to prepare, little people to deliver to school, and, because you are leaving later than usual, you get stuck in traffic. Meanwhile, your mobile phone starts ringing, with people at the office wondering where you are, as you are supposed to be in a meeting, but you are stuck in rush-hour traffic, and your brain has gone into overdrive with the enormity of your morning. And you have only been up for an hour!

When you finally burst through the doors at work, all you can think about is how much you want a coffee. So all morning you have been making adrenalin, and now you are going to make even more adrenalin, as caffeine promotes its production. All you actually want from the coffee at this point in your day is a little breathing space, a moment in time just for you. The reasons we crave a hot drink vary, but without realizing it, sometimes it is just a chance to catch our breath. In those coffee-break moments, it is as though there is a bubble around us, and we are silently communicating, "Don't you dare come near me for the next three minutes!" I have had countless women tell me that coffee is the only peace they get in their day, which, if you look at the reality of it, is not true, as physically coffee is actually adding to the demand on the adrenal glands, pushing them to produce adrenalin to get you away from danger that doesn't actually exist.

There is an important distinction to make between the past and the modern-day. The biochemical changes generated by adrenalin, such as glucose being dumped into your blood to get you out of danger, serve a useful purpose when you are physically fighting or fleeing, but if you are sitting at your desk and sugar is dumped into your blood, you make insulin to deal with that elevation in blood sugar. And insulin is one of our primary fat-storage hormones. Not only that, but it sets your blood sugar up to crash at a later stage, creating a fatigued state that makes you feel like only more caffeine or high-sugar food can fix it. You can already see how adrenalin might make you go for foods or drinks that you know don't serve your well-being. You will also see, in the "Fat Storage, Sugar and Appetite" section in this book, that when you don't utilize the glucose in your blood as fuel it gets stored as glycogen first, and then any left over is stored as body fat.

Caffeine

Consumption Rates

Over 90% of adults in the Western world consume caffeine daily. More than 50% of Americans consume 13 or more caffeinated drinks per week. In Australia and New Zealand, studies suggest that caffeine consumption has more than tripled since the 1960s and, although levels may not be on par with rates of consumption in the United States, they are rapidly rising, not only due to an increase in coffee consumption, but also due to the widespread use of caffeine as an ingredient in, for example, energy drinks. In the United States, 70% of soft drinks contain caffeine. In a US study conducted in 2011, 28% of coffee drinkers had their first cup within 15 minutes of waking and 68% within an hour of waking, while 57% added sugar or sweetener to their brew. The level of caffeine consumption for far too many people is considered addictive by medical textbook standards.

Effect of Caffeine

Here's what happens when you consume caffeine. Caffeine sends a message to the pituitary gland in your brain that it needs to send a message to the adrenal glands to make stress hormones: adrenalin and/or cortisol. When adrenalin is released, your blood sugar elevates to provide you with more energy (ie, fuel); your blood pressure and pulse rate rise to provide more oxygen to the muscles, which tense in preparation for action. Reproductive functions are down-regulated, since they use a lot of energy and are not necessary for your immediate survival, given the impending "threat". Plus, your body does not believe it is safe to bring a baby into what it perceives to be an unsafe world, as adrenalin tells your body that your life is in danger, and cortisol communicates that there is no more food left in the world!

Adrenalin production can be the result of real or perceived stress, or simply the result of your caffeine intake. Caffeine, via stress hormones, and coupled with the signal to activate the fight-or-flight response, fires you up. Once triggered, in this state you have little hope of being calm and centred.

In addition, this biochemical state puts all of its resources into saving your life rather than into what are considered non-vital processes, processes inside you that allow the digestive system and the reproductive system to work optimally, as well as interfering with the nourishment of skin, hair, nails. Over time, the lack of resources available to these non-vital (not necessary to sustain life) processes has significant consequences internally and externally. First, your skin, hair and nails won't receive the nutrients and other substances they need to look their best. Secondly, because the fuel that drives the fight-or-flight response is glucose (ie, sugar), you will crave sugar to constantly refill your fuel tank, and you won't utilize your fat stores often or easily. Also, with additional glucose in your blood, you will release insulin — a fat-storage hormone — and it will first convert unused glucose from your blood into glycogen and store it in your muscles; what is left over will be converted into body fat. Powerful isn't it?

Let me explain this with the story of a client I will call Susan.

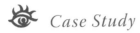

Case Study

Susan's Story

This strikingly slim and physically beautiful woman had an appointment to see me. I did what I do with every client, and asked her how I could help and what she would like to get out of our session. Susan apologized for what she thought would sound vain, and said that she had gained 3 kilograms recently and was seeing me because nothing in her diet or activity level had changed and could be attributed to the weight gain. She was concerned that she may be perimenopausal, even though her periods had not changed. Some of her friends had gained weight during perimenopause, and she was here because she was concerned that those 3 kilograms would become 10 before she knew it, if she didn't get to the bottom of why her body had changed. I admired Susan's attitude and her desire to understand her body better.

We discussed many facets of her life, emotional and physical, and when it came time to talk about her food, her diet was outstanding with regards to all of my benchmarks for eating a diet based on fresh foods. People like me have numerous strategies that we can apply to assist someone on their quest for body fat loss; from a food perspective, this lady was already living that way.

When it came time to talk about her liquid intake, she informed me that she had one glass of red wine four times per week and that she had done this with her husband for years. And then I asked if she drank coffee. Susan's eyes lit up. She replied that, yes, she loved it, but acknowledged, on reflection, that her caffeine intake was something that had changed. She had always had a coffee before breakfast every day for most of her adult life, and that was the only caffeine she consumed all day. But for the past three to four months, she had begun to have up to four coffees per day, but she didn't know why. She just had. When my eyes lit up back at her, she quickly justified her intake by saying, "But they are all black coffees, so there are no calories in them." She drank them all at her desk, she never exercised, and I could see that she had very little muscle mass. Susan herself observed that her fat had gone on around her tummy.

Susan could see from the look on my face where I was about to go and, before I had even spoken, she said, "Please don't take them from me." I wanted her to see how emotionally attached she was to this drink, so I didn't interrupt her. Eventually, I said that I believed it was the coffee that had led to the change in her body, and she cried. She literally cried. That was impossible, she said, and she kept coming back to the calorie reasoning. Basically, she had a tantrum in my office.

I gently tried to lead her to the truth that actually it's only a drink; yet she behaved as though her four daily coffees held the meaning of life for her. I went on to explain the mechanism that I have outlined above involving caffeine, adrenalin, elevated blood sugar, and subsequent insulin production. I told her I wasn't even asking her to give up caffeine entirely, but rather to go back to her one cup a day before breakfast, a coffee prepared with love by her husband, and see what happened.

Susan agreed to make this change for four weeks, even though she couldn't imagine anything being more powerful than calories in body fat creation and so couldn't see how this plan could possibly work. I did nothing else for this woman. Not one other change to her dietary intake, and four weeks later she burst through my door telling me she had lost 4 kilograms in four weeks. She had only gained 3 kilograms in the first place.

As an aside, I have never weighed a client, nor will I ever weigh a client, as I believe you simply weigh your self-esteem when you weigh yourself.

My theory was that Susan's weight gain was the result of stress hormone production from the additional caffeine — and the cascade of effects that this can have, including increased insulin release — rather than the result of too many calories. Her subsequent weight loss was, in my opinion, extremely fast, but my point in sharing this story is to demonstrate caffeine's power to signal what is, for some, fat storage, and also its ability to create an almost crazed emotional state, demonstrated by Susan's tantrum when we first met. Decreasing her coffee consumption seemed like an overwhelming task for Susan, but she stuck with it and reaped the benefits.

Such fast weight loss will not happen for everyone, but the level of calm and well-being certainly improves with less caffeine. Weight loss significantly depends on the balance between your sympathetic and your parasympathetic nervous systems, as explained in the "Red Zone Green Zone" section. You really want to get your head around that concept as well.

It is so important that you consider your caffeine habits and get honest with yourself about how it affects you. Does it dull your appetite, and so unconsciously you grab a coffee instead of eating? This is especially true for many women at lunchtime. Does it make your heart race, give you the shakes, or loosen your bowels? Does it elevate your blood pressure? Do you notice you want it more when you are stressed, and, if so, what story have you attached to what coffee gives you? Do you have restless, poor-quality sleep because of how much caffeine you consume? Or does it lift your mood or nourish your soul with no ill effect whatsoever? My clients will tell you that, when it is warranted, I ask them to give up caffeine completely for a four-week trial period. They are often shocked by how much more energy they have without caffeine in their lives, not to mention having less or no anxiety! You know yourself better than anyone. Act on what you know is true for you.

> *It is so important that you consider your caffeine habits.*

A Little Note on Tea

Not so long ago, tea was the major source of caffeine for people in Australia and New Zealand, before the coffee culture hit town. Tea contains caffeine, although how much depends on how long you brew it. An average cup of black tea contains 50 milligrams of caffeine, whereas green tea tends to contain about 30 milligrams per cup. Tea, however, also contains another substance called *theanine*, which acts as an antioxidant but also helps buffer the effect of the caffeine. It makes you alert but not wired. Some people are actually highly caffeine-sensitive, and even green tea can impact them negatively. However, many people tolerate tea and feel good drinking tea compared with coffee. They may not realize this until they take a break from coffee, though.

The Pace of Life

Think about all of these mechanisms. So many people run on adrenalin these days. Moment to moment, day to day, it is as though a light-switch has gone on, and it hasn't entirely switched off for a really long time. And it doesn't have to be traumatic stress and/or shocking situations that drive this process. It can simply be the pace at which we live our lives: being contactable 24/7; constant exposure to social media, unless we purposefully choose otherwise; the juggling act that leads so many people I meet, women in particular, to say that they want more "balance" in their lives, as they can't cope like this anymore. (I wrote *Rushing Woman's Syndrome* for women who feel like this, and to guide them out of the rush.)

The human body is incredibly resilient and, although we were not designed to withstand long-term stress (due to the way we are designed, we are healthier when it is short-lived), many bodies appear to tolerate, but not necessarily thrive on, years and years of living on adrenalin. Yet I have witnessed first-hand what the relentless production of this hormone does to women's health, including its impact on their fertility, the incidence and severity of premenstrual syndrome (PMS), their digestive systems, their skin, their relationships, their happiness, and the shape and size of their body. An additional challenge, however, is that once the body perceives that the stress has become long-term, your dominant stress hormone can begin to change, and that can have significant consequences on your metabolism.

Cortisol — Friend or Worst Nightmare?

Cortisol is your long-term (ie, chronic) stress hormone. Historically, the only long-term stress humans had revolved around food being scarce. Long-term stress came in the form of floods, famines and wars. During such times, a person didn't know where the next meal was coming from. Today, in the Western world, our long-term stresses tend to be based more on financial situations, relationship concerns, challenges with friendships, particularly for teenage girls, and uncertainty or worries about our health or bodies. I can't tell you how many times I have heard women say that they would "do anything" for a different body part — thinner thighs, less body hair, no cellulite — and for many women the part or parts of themselves that they dislike intensely become a silent fixation in their minds. For so many women, their first waking thoughts involve "What will I, or won't I, eat today?" or "How much exercise can I get done today?"

So many women rush through their days with a pervasive not-good-enough or never-enough-time monologue running through their head. Day after day, this can easily lead to a chronic pattern of stress response, hence increased cortisol output. In turn, this can lead to a significant change in your metabolism and where you store fat on your body.

How Cortisol Works

It is important to understand how cortisol works, as it can be your friend or one of your worst nightmares. When made at optimum amounts, cortisol does numerous wonderful things for your health. It is one of the body's primary anti-inflammatory mediators, meaning that wherever there is inflammation in the body, which is a process involved in most disease states, cortisol, having been converted into cortisone, dampens down the effect of that inflammation and stops your body from feeling stiff, rigid or in pain. Many people, for example, describe feeling that they have suddenly aged as they come out of difficult times, and often this is the result of sub-optimal cortisol levels during such periods. In the right amount, cortisol is not only an anti-inflammatory, it also buffers the effect of insulin, meaning that optimum amounts of cortisol help you continue to burn body fat for energy while also maintaining stable (as opposed to rapidly fluctuating) blood sugar levels.

Cortisol levels change over the day. The right amount at the right time assists you with various bodily functions throughout the course of the day. Cortisol is designed to be high in the morning and, for the purpose of this discussion, let's say that 25 units at around 6am are ideal. Cortisol is one of the mechanisms that wake you up in the morning and help you bounce out of bed full of energy and vitality, rather than snooze an hour away and still end up feeling like you have been hit by a truck. By midday, optimum cortisol will sit at around 15 units, and, by 6pm, levels will ideally be at around 4 units. By 10pm, optimum cortisol levels are around two units, a level at which they are designed to stay until around 2am, when they slowly and very steadily begin to rise again.

So it is true what your mother told you — that one hour of sleep before midnight is worth two after.

The following graph illustrates this. So it is true what your mother told you — that one hour of sleep before midnight is worth two after — because cortisol starts to rise around 2am and the waking-up process gradually begins.

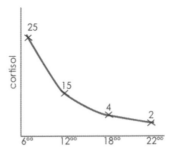

The optimal cortisol profile: Cortisol is nice and high in the morning, and falls away again by the evening.

As a stress response continues, its effect on the body begins to change. In the early stages of stress, one of the first challenges cortisol presents is that the evening level of the hormone starts to spike again rather than continue to decrease. At this stage, you still make optimum levels in the morning and are able to bounce out of bed and get on with your day with reasonable energy, but evening levels are creeping up. This is one mechanism through which good sleeping patterns can be interrupted. Research has shown that enough good-quality sleep is another factor critical for weight loss.

When cortisol levels become elevated above optimal, other changes in body chemistry begin to unfold. It has been suggested that elevated cortisol is the one common thread behind what we have come to describe as *metabolic syndrome*; that is, elevated blood pressure, elevated cholesterol, and insulin resistance. This last condition is a warning sign that, if nothing changes in the near future, type 2 diabetes is a likely consequence.

It is important to remember that we are completely geared for survival, and that elevated cortisol tells every cell of our body that food is scarce. This means that one of its roles is to slow down your metabolic rate. Cortisol's concern is that if you keep utilizing energy at a more rapid rate, you may become too thin and die. So it slows down our metabolism and tells your body to store fat, not burn it, in an attempt to put some more flesh on your bones so you are more likely to survive the famine your body perceives you are facing.

One of the ways cortisol slows down your metabolic rate is by breaking down your muscles. Cortisol is what is known as a *catabolic hormone*. It breaks body proteins down into their building blocks, known as *amino acids,* and with less muscle mass, you burn fewer calories. Your muscles, for example, are made from proteins, and cortisol signals them to break down, as the body's perception is that fuel is needed. Additional amino acids are also needed in the blood to help repair tissues from this chronic stress you are enduring, even though you may be simply sitting on your bottom in front of the television, with your financial or relationship concerns milling around in your head. The amino acids released as a result of the catabolic signalling of cortisol can be converted, through a process called *gluconeogenesis,* back into glucose (sugar), which your body thinks may be useful to assist you in your stress. Yet, if you are not active, this increase in blood glucose will not be utilized, and insulin will have to be secreted to return blood glucose levels to normal by returning the glucose in the blood to storage. Remember that glucose is stored as glycogen in the muscles and the liver.

Over time, the catabolic signalling of cortisol itself may have broken down some of your muscles, so now there is less space for glucose storage. As a result, some of the blood glucose returns to the remaining muscles while the leftovers are converted into body fat. Keeping the glucose level of the blood within the normal, safe range is of more importance to your body than whether you have wobbly bits around your middle! Essentially, too much cortisol can make you fat through dysregulated blood sugar metabolism, not just fat metabolism itself. This is one of the mechanisms through which cellulite can appear, as where muscles once were, fat can now be deposited. This is also the process through which long-term stress can contribute to type 2 diabetes.

Because excess cortisol is produced after the stress in your life has been going on for a while, your body — not knowing any better — thinks there is no more food left in your world, and it instinctively knows that it has a greater chance of survival if it holds onto some extra body fat. In modern times, when, for health reasons or vanity (or both), many people understand the importance of not carrying too much body fat, cortisol can provide a potential challenge to someone who believes that eating less (ie, a diet) is their only solution to body fat loss. Yet if you eat less when excess cortisol is already telling your body that there is no food left in the world, you will confirm to your body what it perceives is true — that there is no food left in the world — and your metabolism will be slowed even further. Feeling like you are fighting an uphill battle with your body can be an immense source of stress, adding another layer of stress to an already busy life. It can also lead people to feel like their body is betraying them, for throughout this metabolic change they may (or not) be making great efforts with food and movement. In other words, they may be ensuring their calorie equation is skewed for weight loss, but they are not achieving this. If anything, their clothes continue to fit them the way they have for a while or they become tighter, despite great efforts. This alone can be incredibly disheartening. Going on a diet is never the right medicine.

Understanding the Cortisol Problem

If cortisol tells every cell of your body that food is scarce, and your metabolism slows down as a result, and you continue to eat and exercise in the same way you always have, your clothes will slowly get tighter. In this situation, as far as body fat loss goes, it doesn't matter how amazingly you eat; with cortisol telling every cell in your body to store fat, it is very difficult, if not impossible, to decrease body fat until the cortisol issue is resolved. We must get to the heart of the stress and either change the situation or change the perception. That doesn't mean you give up on taking care of how you nourish your body, though. It needs all of the nutrients it can get, even more so when there is stress. Just remember that focusing on the calorie equation — how much you eat versus how much you move — won't solve a waistline that is expanding due to elevated cortisol.

Cortisol has a distinct fat deposition pattern. If cortisol is an issue for you, you typically lay it on around your tummy, and once again the reason for fat placement here is governed by the body's quest for survival. If food suddenly did run out, your major organs have easy access to fat that will keep you alive. You also tend to lay down fat on the back of the arms (you get "bingo wings"), and you grow what I lovingly call a back verandah. So what do most people do when they notice that their clothes are getting tighter? They go on a diet, which typically means eating less. Eating less, though, just confirms to your body what it perceives to be true — that food is scarce — and so slows down your metabolism even further. But food is not scarce; it is abundant for you. If you want a chocolate bar at 3am, you can get one.

Another challenge you face with elevated cortisol is that, since your body thinks that food is scarce, any time you see food it is very easy to over-eat. No matter how firmly you intend to eat only three crackers when you get home from work, if that open packet of crackers is in front of you, cortisol will scream at every cell of your body: "You are so lucky! There's food here — eat it!" And somehow, before you know it, the whole box of crackers is gone. Don't get me wrong: I am not saying that self-discipline and willpower have no place. You could make a decision right now that, when it comes to what you put into your body, from this point forward you are going to raise your standards. You could do that right now. My intention in explaining this is simply to point out that humans have very ancient hormonal mechanisms at work inside their bodies that believe they know better than your conscious mind when it comes to your survival. Your body can be your biggest teacher if you learn how to decipher its messages. Extra body fat, or whichever body part you focus on and wish you could change, are sometimes simply vehicles of communication, asking you to explore your biochemistry and the beliefs that have led to this situation. In *Beauty from the Inside Out* I phrased this "The parts of your body that frustrate or sadden you are simply messengers asking you to eat, drink, move, think, believe or perceive in a new way. See them as the gift that they are."

Guilt and cortisol

When you feel grateful for the life you have, it is easy to feel guilty if you complain about anything. A common internal phrase might be "There are so many people worse off than me." Such thinking immediately makes you feel guilty, and you stop focusing on your source of stress. Trouble is, although there *are* people worse off than you in this world, the minute you feel guilty you change your focus so that you don't ever get the opportunity to identify what is bothering you, and more importantly why. What is bothering you can offer an insightful road in to the core of something bigger, if you follow it with curiosity.

Many women keep the peace to avoid stress. Yet there is no peace when you have to keep the peace. Think about that. Here is a common example to help you see how everyday life, because of the perceptions we bring to it, can lead to cortisol, from an emotional source, being a contributor to health challenges.

Basic psychology teaches us that humans will do more to avoid pain than they will ever do to experience pleasure. Some women I meet will do anything, for example, to keep the peace and avoid conflict. Inwardly, they become highly strung because they are always walking on eggshells around others, especially their intimate partner, doing all they can to help prevent those around them from losing their temper. If the man of the house has a tendency to communicate with explosive, angry outbursts that seem unpredictable — hello, silent stress hormone production!

Some women avoid feeling emotional pain by eating too much or making other poor food choices; perhaps drinking bucket-loads of wine or chain-smoking cigarettes. Some go shopping and rack up credit-card bills that will take months or years to pay off. Alternatively, some people might cope or explore their pain by writing in a journal, or going for a walk or a swim. Others will pray, meditate, or telephone a friend and chat to deal with emotional pain. Some of the ways we cope with or explore what is going on support our health. Some potentially harm our health. And all of these activities may take place with or without a conscious understanding of why.

I want to help you see *why*, so that you can change your response, if it is hurting your health, especially if the stress hormone production triggered by your subconscious emotional responses is blocking you from experiencing the amazing human that you are.

Worrying and weight gain

As we now know, stress — whether it is real or perceived — may promote the production of excess cortisol. The ripple effect of constant worries can slowly and subtly change your metabolism to one of fat storage, leave your headspace full of sadness, and cause you to withdraw and fly off the handle in frustration at things that don't warrant such a reaction. What is driving this are the chemical signals created by your body, which it believes will help you, based on the information it is receiving.

I love this quote by Marcus Aurelius, which may assist you if worry is a pattern for you: "If you are troubled by external circumstances, it is not the circumstances that trouble you, but your own perception of them — and they are in your power to change at any time." Do something creative with that quote — stick it on your fridge if it helps.

Adrenal Fatigue

The next biochemical stage of stress that can occur, especially if the stress has been prolonged, may involve cortisol levels falling low, and these days I see more and more of this in younger and younger people. If you have had a high level of cortisol output for many, many years, your adrenal glands may not be able to sustain this. They are not designed to withstand this kind of output, and so they crash. In general terms, you burn out. Your energy crashes. In more recent times, this has become known as *adrenal fatigue*, because the major symptom is a deep, unrelenting fatigue.

Yet even with fatigue as the major symptom, what I have observed over the past decade is that not only are people beyond tired, at the same time they can also be wired, although not always. And when you are tired but wired, you desire deeply restorative sleep more than ever, yet it rarely happens; your adrenal hormone production is usually at the heart of this. The pituitary gland in your brain regulates your adrenals (and the rest of your endocrine system), and, although treatment for adrenal fatigue usually involves a range of strategies that support the adrenals themselves, going one step further and assisting the pituitary gland can also be immensely powerful and highly beneficial to restoring your health and vitality. In my opinion, a form of yoga known as Restorative Yoga, or Stillness Through Movement, is the most effective way to make progress in recovering from adrenal fatigue.

As you now understand, the adrenal hormone cortisol is supposed to be high in the morning, helping you to bounce out of bed. It plays a role in how vital you feel and helps the body combat any inflammatory processes that

> *The pituitary gland in your brain regulates your adrenals.*

want to kick in. Stiffness is a key symptom of adrenal fatigue. For those with chronic stress, morning cortisol levels tend to be low; if 25 units is the ideal, with adrenal stress you may only get to 10 units, or even less. It can be very difficult to get out of bed with such low levels. By mid-afternoon it will be at an all-time low, and you will usually feel you need something sweet and/or something containing caffeine, and/or a nap to get you through your afternoon. (This can also be the result of low blood sugar or poor thyroid function, explored in other sections.) For an adrenally fatigued person, cortisol is nice and low in the evenings, as it is supposed to be. But, if you don't go to bed before 10pm, you will typically get a second wind, and it will be much harder for you to fall asleep if you are still up at midnight, partly due to the body's natural next adrenalin surge (not cortisol) that tends to happen between 10.30pm and 11.30pm. The following graph illustrates this cortisol pattern.

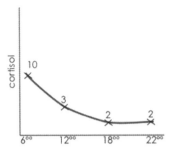

A typical cortisol profile of an adrenally fatigued person: Note, particularly, the low waking cortisol and low midday reading.

When cortisol drops low, it is likely that prior to this it was high (although not always) and body fat may have increased during this time. But just because cortisol is low does not necessarily mean easy access to body fat burning, due to cortisol's relationship to insulin, as described earlier. Plus if cortisol was previously high, your muscle mass will likely be less, and as a result your metabolism slower than it was previously, before the stress began.

Additionally, the fatigue you feel with this biochemical picture may make exercise the least appealing thing on the planet to you. You actually tend to feel worse after exercise when you are adrenally fatigued, whereas exercise typically energizes. When we are sedentary some enzymes necessary for fat-burning aspects of metabolism are down-regulated, too. Frustration mounts because, like most people in the Western world, you have probably believed that exercising and eating less are the only solutions to weight loss, yet you can't bring yourself to do either despite every good intention. You eat something sweet, or consume highly processed carbohydrates in desperate search of energy, or you eat too much, or another month goes past without much movement ... And when you reflect on this, you feel guilty, you might say mean things to yourself, and you may silently lose hope. Your clothes keep getting tighter, and this just adds to your stress. You can see how this vicious cycle can be self-perpetuating.

Humans were never designed to sustain long-term stress,

and our individual bodies cope with it in different ways. For some, adrenalin remains the dominant stress hormone all of their lives, while others may flip over into a more cortisol-dominant stress response. If the stress response doesn't truly switch off, there is the potential that the adrenals will eventually crash, and cortisol output is no longer optimum or elevated; it will be negligible. At its extreme, this can become a condition called Addison's disease. Yet if a person's cortisol level is extremely low but still falls just inside the "normal range", they will be told that they are fine. They may feel lousy, but all the tests they have always come back "normal". They feel anything but normal, and people who know and love them will often comment that they are a shell of their former selves.

Cortisol can also be rather sinister in that it can interfere with your steroid (sex) hormone metabolism, sleep patterns, your mood, insulin and blood glucose management, as well as thyroid function, all elements that influence metabolism — and that the calorie equation does not consider.

A Typical Stress Pattern in Adulthood

Something you weren't expecting happens: you lose your job, a relationship suddenly ends and you didn't want it to, someone you love passes away. Adrenalin production kicks in. You feel like you are in shock. You lose weight without trying. If the stress or the ramifications of the stress continue, your body can't sustain the output of adrenalin and all of its biochemical consequences (inflammation, for example). With the continuing stress, your body has no choice but to start to make more cortisol than before. You gain weight. It doesn't seem to matter how little you eat or how often you exercise, nothing changes. You have thickened up through the middle and it won't seem to budge. With the ongoing stress you tend to drink alcohol each evening to avoid feeling the emotional pain, and so you wake up tired and start every day with coffee to get your self going; two liver-loaders. This adds to the stress inside your body, and over the long term can disrupt sex hormone balance and lead to fat accumulation in the liver, with energy continuing to decline and body fat continuing to increase.

No diet will resolve this. Resolving the emotional pain will. Resolving why you have stopped seeing and treating yourself as the precious human you are, will.

Stressed and Skinny

There are people who are very stressed and their weight doesn't fluctuate. Some people who are stressed are too slim and find it difficult to gain weight, and many are highly frustrated by this. Not everyone's body responds in the same way to stress. There are other metabolic factors at play with the different stress hormones, so you want to treat what *your* body is communicating to you.

Don't Sweat the Small Stuff

One thing I have observed (not based on scientific research, this is an observation) is that certain people are what I call "emotional cruisers". They are genuinely quite laid-back, they don't sweat the small stuff. Whether they were born this way or have learnt to be so from going through some big things in life, they truly don't sweat the small stuff. Deep in their hearts they know and trust that it is all OK, that it is all part of a bigger picture, that life happens for you, not to you, *and* they eat mostly real food — 90% or more of the time. Consequently, their weight is far more stable. This is why in my work — through books, seminars and weekend events — my intention is to support people in finding a way that serves their individual needs with food *and* their beliefs.

Strategies for Adrenal Support

The Importance of Rest

At the heart of all of my strategies to support you adrenally so that you can experience amazing health, as well as use body fat effectively, is the desire for you to rest and to rest well, in a restorative and revitalizing way. Rest must follow action, for us to have optimal health, excellent fat burning, the ability to remain calm, and all those "non-vital" processes mentioned earlier, such as our skin, hair, and nails getting all the nourishment they need. And very few of us these days truly rest or live in a calm state, where productivity, patience, and kindness tend to easily flow.

The nervous system was explored at length in a previous section. Remember the PNS — the rest, digest, repair and reproduce arm of the nervous system; the green zone? It is critical to remember that appropriate activation of the PNS is essential not only to our fat utilization, but also to feeling centred and calm, and having a tummy that isn't bloated after eating. Food is not supposed to bloat us, yet a bloated stomach is a major complaint for one in five women in Australia and New Zealand. Calm is vital to optimal digestion. I have received countless emails from women who have taken my advice to focus on chewing well, on eating slowly, and on eating more real food, who, after even three days, no longer bloat. Imagine that. This happens because:

⊕ eating like this, instead of inhaling food, slows down or stops stress hormone production, allowing the blood supply to support the digestive system

⊕ chewing food well stimulates stomach acid and digestive enzymes, enhancing digestion

⊕ the body knows how to digest real food.

The Importance of Diaphragmatic Breathing

Breathing is the only way we can consciously affect our autonomic nervous system (ANS), the part of the nervous system from where the red and green zones stem. We cannot control our ANS with our thoughts; we cannot instruct it what to do. How we breathe is our only road in there. Every time I write or say that out loud, I am reminded of just how magical and miraculous the human body is.

The impact of diaphragmatic breathing on the nervous

system is one of the main reasons why it is the cornerstone of all my adrenal support solutions. If you take nothing else away from this book, I would like to encourage you with every ounce of my being to incorporate a ritual into your day that allows you to focus on breathing diaphragmatically. It is key to shifting our chemistry from fat storage to fat burning.

How can the breath drive such powerful shifts in your nervous system and your biochemistry? The role of the ANS is to perceive the external environment and, after processing the information in the central nervous system, regulate the function of your internal environment. The name *autonomic* implies that it is independent of the conscious mind. Think about a family of ducks and their newborn ducklings. Just like ducklings, the autonomic nervous system will always follow the leader, and the breath is the *only* part of the autonomic nervous system that can be controlled consciously. Your breath leads. Your body follows. Breathing dominates your autonomic nervous system, and because we breathe 5000 to 30,000 times a day — or 200 million to 500 million times in a lifetime — it has the potential to

> *N*othing communicates to every cell of your body that you are safe better than diaphragmatic breathing.

influence us positively, or negatively, in many ways.

Nothing communicates to every cell of your body that you are safe better than diaphragmatic breathing. If you breathe in a shallow way, with short, sharp inhalations and exhalations, then you are communicating to your body via your ANS that your life is in danger. Remember the cascade of hormonal events that follow such an alarm, and the role these hormones play, for one thing, in switching fat burning on or off.

How you breathe can also be a fast-track to the symptoms of anxiety, and potentially panic attacks, regardless of what led you to breathe in a shallow way in the first place. Whether it was an event, a deadline, the perception of pressure, the "need" to rush, or the lifetime habit of your nervous system, the result is the same. Long, slow breathing that moves your diaphragm communicates the opposite message to your body — that you are very safe. Nothing down-regulates the production of fat-storage stress hormones or the alarm signals within your body more powerfully. No practice restores your vitality like regularly breathing this way. And I don't say that lightly.

Practise diaphragmatic breathing, making sure your tummy moves in and out as you breathe, as opposed to just your upper chest. You can begin your breath by allowing the lower part of your tummy to expand, and then imagine as the breath slowly continues that the expansion of your tummy has now extended into the area where you can feel it meet your ribcage. Keep the slow inhalation going until your upper chest feels like it is pushing your ribs out at the sides of your body. Then pause, rather than hold your breath, and slowly allow the exhalation to begin in the reverse order of the inhalation, with the top and side of the chest emptying first, followed by the middle of your abdomen and lastly your tummy. If that sounds or feels too tricky, just move your tummy (abdomen) in and out with each breath, allow it to expand on the inhale and shrink back in on the exhale.

Be kind and patient with yourself, as this takes practice! You may feel like you are unable to get parts of your body to engage at first, but in time and with practice the parts of you that have become disconnected will be thrilled to be back in touch.

At first, you will more than likely need to schedule regular diaphragmatic breathing time slots into your day until it becomes your new way of breathing. Make appointments with yourself to breathe in this way. If it is peaceful each morning while you boil the kettle for the first time that day (to make your hot water with lemon, of course), instead of racing around and doing 80 jobs while the kettle boils, stand in your kitchen and breathe. Link breathing well to a daily routine, such as having a shower, or to a particular hour of the day, so that it quickly becomes a habit. Do it numerous times over the course of your day. Book a meeting into your calendar each afternoon at 3pm. If you work at a computer, have it pop up on the screen that it is time for your meeting with yourself to do 20 long, slow breaths. We keep appointments with other people, so be sure to keep the appointments you make with yourself.

Take part in movement that facilitates a focus on the breath, such as t'ai chi, qigong, yoga, particularly restorative yoga, or walking quietly in Nature. Pilates can also be useful, but I have found that it is highly dependent on your attitude while you are doing the session, and also to some degree on the attitude of the instructor. For me personally, qigong is the main way I choose to begin my day. I had a period of time where I let this ritual go, and I learnt very quickly how crucial it is to set up my day with a restoration-focused session. Without it, my clarity, my sex hormone balance, and my vitality are not what I know they can be. So, please, schedule breath-focused periods into your day, and keep your appointments with yourself. Breathing is the cornerstone PNS activation which means great energy, vitality, calm and readily burnt body fat. These practices allow us to still the stories, still the monkey mind, which can be one of the sources of daily stress.

The Importance of Laughter

Another free and powerful tool is laughter. If we see life as tough, and full of hard work, pain and drudgery, it will be precisely that. Humans have the ability to see only their perspective in the world, rather than the world as it truly is. We see the world through filters, even though we often don't know they are there. I am not denying that life can be tough at times, or that being honest with ourselves if we do feel down and out about life is a good thing. The problem comes when we see the world this way and believe that it will never be any different. For then it won't be.

Think about it. A belief in the permanence of doom is dangerous for every hormonal signal in your body. Do your absolute best to shift your thinking to see life as an adventure, a journey, a gift full of opportunity, and a process through which you can contribute. Some of the greatest, most moving stories I have ever heard involved someone turning a horrific hardship into their greatest opportunity, and a way to give back. Keep this in mind. Keep in mind, too, that you can choose to laugh at the calamity around you. I remember clearly witnessing this when my dearest friend had her third baby, and, with him not even a day old, countless well-wishers chattering away, a hospital staff member wanting to clear the food tray away, and her deliciously spirited two-year-old daughter not being too thrilled about this as she wanted the remaining apple juice — and all in one small room — my precious friend and her husband just shrugged and grinned at each other and laughed, internally clearly focused on the love in the room, rather than on anything else. What you focus on is what you feel.

> Do your absolute best to shift your thinking to see life as an adventure, a journey, a gift full of opportunity.

◈ Can Stress Increase Body Fat? In Short ...

Adrenalin:

- ◈ is your acute stress hormone
- ◈ drives the fight-or-flight response
- ◈ communicates to every cell in your body that your life is in danger
- ◈ needs to fuel you to get out of danger fast, therefore promotes the utilization of fast-burning glucose as a fuel, as opposed to slow-burning fat
- ◈ can lead to insulin resistance as it leads to the constant release of glucose from the liver and muscles — if this glucose isn't utilized in escaping (exercise/movement), insulin has to be made to take it back to storage, and some of it will likely be stored as fat
- ◈ diverts blood away from your digestive system to your arms and legs to power you to get out of danger, therefore digestion is compromised
- ◈ because it communicates that your life is in danger, it interferes with the body's ability to make optimal amounts of progesterone, a sex hormone involved in fertility and a hormone that acts as an anti-anxiety agent, an antidepressant and a diuretic — if adrenalin stops efficient progesterone production, this is one way a woman can become oestrogen-dominant, which leads to additional fat storage
- ◈ doesn't tend to lead people to gain weight directly; some studies suggest it speeds up metabolism preparing you to fight or run — the problem is your body can't sustain the output as adrenalin increases blood pressure and promotes inflammation (among other processes), the basis of all degenerative diseases in the body
- ◈ if the output is sustained, the body can't withstand the biochemical changes that the adrenalin drives, so the body starts to make extra cortisol to help combat these changes (as, for example, cortisol is an anti-inflammatory).

Cortisol:

- ◆ does good things for health when it is made in the right amount: it is an anti-inflammatory, modulates the insulin response, and is an important immune system regulator
- ◆ is your chronic stress hormone: while typically long-term stress for humans was floods, famines and wars, today it tends to be worry about finances, relationships, health, and the health of a loved one; because historically the chronic stress situations typically meant food was scarce, cortisol communicates to the body that food is scarce
- ◆ is catabolic, meaning it breaks your muscles down
- ◆ slows your metabolic rate
- ◆ lays fat down around the tummy, the back of the arms and you grow "a back verandah", because the body perceives there is no food left in the world, and all of the vital organs that keep you alive (except for your brain) are housed in your torso, so they need protection, warmth and nutrients to get through the "famine"
- ◆ is believed to be one of the hormones at the heart of metabolic syndrome, when it is in excess for too long
- ◆ can interfere with sex hormone balance, as it communicates to your body that there is no food left in the world so the last thing a woman's body wants for her when she is churning out stress hormones is to bring a baby into a world where the body perceives it is not safe (adrenalin) and where there is no food (cortisol)
- ◆ can disrupt thyroid function through a variety of mechanisms
- ◆ can impede restorative sleep
- ◆ might not be made in large enough amounts after long periods of chronic stress — if this occurs, it is referred to as "adrenal fatigue", where morning waking cortisol is particularly low; if the body can't make enough cortisol, then inflammation and fatigue, as well as additional disruption to other endocrine glands, can ensue.

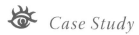 *Case Study*

Mrs J's story

Mrs J was a 48-year-old woman who saw me for weight loss. She had been eating a low-fat, low-calorie diet (1280–1400 per day) and exercising at the gym five days a week, doing cardio classes for seven months. She said she was fed up with it all, as she had lost no weight or body fat at all. The gym had weighed her when she signed up, and had taken her body fat measurements, and repeated this at the three- and six-month marks. Her body fat started at 33%, went to 34%, and then back to 33%, across each time point.

On further questioning, I found out that Mrs J was highly stressed due to a long-term, ongoing family situation she could not change. She had seen a psychologist about this previously. Her additional body fat was primarily on her torso, rather than on her arms and legs. She said she did not sleep well, and had previously used alcohol to fall asleep, but had stopped drinking, except for one glass on a Friday night, since she started her diet and exercise regime. However, she still woke up a lot during the night. Her menstrual cycle was regular, but her blood loss had decreased. She was very red in the face, and said her face flushed easily.

Course of action
Based on her symptoms, I felt Mrs J needed adrenal and liver support, and to overhaul how she was eating. The plan of action I created for Mrs J involved dietary and lifestyle changes, nutritional supplementation and herbal medicine. Keep in mind that what works for one person does not always work for another, so I share this with you only to show you how dietary modification and herbal medicine can make a significant difference.

Dietary changes

- Real food
- No refined (processed) food
- Increased dietary fat, particularly essential fats
- No caffeine, preservatives, additives, colourings or refined sugars
- High plant intake, with good serves of dietary proteins, fat from whole foods, and carbohydrates from whole foods such as sweet potato (kumara), pumpkin and potato

Supplements

Some of the nutrients were combined into one tablet, but I will list the nutrients separately so that you can see what was included.

- Vitamin C
- Magnesium, calcium, vitamin D
- Food-based essential fatty acid supplement
- Food-based green drink supplement

Herbal medicine

Herbal medicines are best tailored to the individual. Mrs J's tonic included herbs to lower cortisol and support phase 2 liver detoxification.

Lifestyle and emotions

- Relaxation through breathing, reading and walking in Nature
- Prioritizing sleep: a minimum of 8 hours per night, and in bed asleep by 10pm
- Changing the gym exercise to resistance training and yoga (instead of cardio), given that she already had a gym membership
- Sticking a copy of the "Serenity Prayer" on the fridge to remind her of its wisdom, given her family situation: "God grant me the serenity to accept the things I cannot change,

courage to change the things I can, and the wisdom to know the difference."

Three months later
Mrs J was a calmer, leaner version of herself. She said she could tell she had lost weight, but had stopped focusing on that or letting the gym weigh her, as she was more concerned with how she felt each day. She reported that she was sleeping through most nights now, which she felt was "life-changing". She decided to have her body fat measured before coming to see me, as she was curious about what that would show, given her clothes were finally looser. Her body fat was 27%. She was thrilled, as that confirmed for her that — coupled with how she was feeling and coping with her life — she was heading in the right direction. She said she could not believe that she could stop doing such intense exercise and eat more total food, especially fat, and get this outcome. She said it made no sense to how she thought the body worked, but she was ecstatic with the outcome.

As an aside, and on a personal note for me, I have wanted to write this book for at least a decade, to debunk the concept that body shape and size is entirely the result of the calorie equation, as I have seen thousands of clients, like Mrs J, over the years in precisely this situation. My clients know that my focus for them has always been to stop dieting and start nourishing, and to provide their individual body with what it needs to be its best, healthy self.

A Few Reasons Why Diets Don't Work

There is a definition of insanity that suggests that doing the same thing over and over, year after year, and expecting a different outcome is crazy. And I agree. No place is this more obvious than with diets. It can feel as though you are in a trance for 10 or 30 years, or, for some, a lifetime, doing all you can to make yourself better, or slimmer, or something that you perceive you are not — given too many people's inherent belief that they aren't enough the way they are. And when you believe you aren't enough, you will never feel like you have enough. Whether your thing is food or clothes or shoes or wine, you will never have enough because you believe you aren't enough.

We can't see that we just keep doing the same thing over and over and our lives never seem to look any different. We think we just require a different diet, or a different exercise programme, or thinner thighs, and that will make all the difference. What people need is insight into what drives their behaviour and then to stop dieting.

It is well-known that the majority of people who go on diets end up regaining any weight they lose plus more — 83% in fact — and they regain it within a two-year period. At the heart of this effect is a precise scientific process which on the surface may appear harmless, yet underneath it is a yo-yo cycle that bounces between strict deprivation and a free-for-all with food. If people try to lose weight by shaming and depriving themselves, weight loss will not necessarily occur; they simply end up ashamed and deprived, and no one can sustain that.

As you now know, biochemically there is a stress hormone called cortisol that the adrenal glands make. Historically, humans only made cortisol in times of physical stress where food was scarce, such as floods, famines and wars. People with the highest levels of body fat tended to survive these times, so cortisol acted to slow down the metabolic rate and communicate to the body that it needed to store fat. Even though we live in a modern world, our subconscious biochemical reactions to chronic stress are the same as they have always been; and even though we may think differently, our subconscious mind, which runs our lives most of the time, is a million times more powerful than our conscious mind.

Over the past two decades, the human body has been asked to change at a rate greater than at any other time in history; a rate I have come to call "Google speed". With the advent of the internet, cellphones, email and social media, we are amped up and on-call 24/7, unless we choose to disconnect. Today, chronic stress, and hence cortisol production, tends to come from long-term psychological worries about relationships, finances, health issues, or body shape, size and weight. We have forgotten how essential it is to every aspect of our health, including our body size, to just switch off, rest, and activate vital restorative processes.

We also tend to make cortisol when we "starve" ourselves. If you suddenly go from over-eating food to not eating very much food at all, your body tends to make cortisol because it doesn't understand that you have just embarked on a diet. It thinks there is no food left in the world so it has no choice but to try to save your life, and to do this it slows your metabolism right down. So then when you stop dieting and you return to the way you used to eat, which you will unless you have truly explored what is at the heart of your matter, you will not just return to the size you once were, you will naturally grow beyond that as your metabolism will have slowed down.

Many people attempt to address this by exercising fanatically, yet when you do this, your body interprets this as fleeing from danger and subconsciously activates the message that it is caught up in the "floods, famines and war" scenario, receiving the biochemical message that to be "safe" it still needs to store fat rather than burn it.

What do most people do when their clothes get tight? They

go on a what? A diet. And when you go on a diet, do you eat more or less? Usually less. Yet when you do this, you simply confirm what your body perceives to be true (what cortisol is communicating): that there is limited food left in the world, when in fact food is likely to be abundant for you.

With any system that addresses weight, unless it also explores what is literally at the heart of someone's situation rather than the size of their thighs, it won't work. Any diet that leads to an initial weight loss that is regained when the diet stops is not a successful diet. I meet people every day who say the X diet worked for them. Yet there they are in front of me physically bigger than they were before they went on the X diet, so, no, actually the X diet did not work for them. If someone has gone on a diet, lost weight, and kept it off, a far deeper shift has happened within them to foster that sustained change.

Because guess what — and what I am about to say may surprise you coming from a nutrition expert — it is not about the food.

The process, life itself, is the goal, not some number that weighs your self-esteem far more than anything else.

At the heart of any addiction, whether that is an addiction to food itself or simply an addiction to constantly judging yourself based on the size and shape of your body, regardless of its shape and size, is the belief in your own deficiency and the assumption that it can be fixed with an external substance or regime.

People eat unresourcefully for many reasons. It can be a biochemical reason, such as low blood glucose, that leads someone to polish off too many sweet foods for afternoon tea, or it can be emotional, such as when someone feels rejected when a colleague gives them constructive feedback, and they try to block the pain of this perceived rejection by eating. Or it can be both. Often it is both.

So now you can truly appreciate part of why diets don't work, due to both biochemical and emotional factors. Despite the latest fad being touted as the ultimate weight-loss solution, they simply offer short-term results for a long-term additional gain. Lasting weight loss is never achieved with a fad that starves your body and your soul, and you miss out on life in the process. When your brain is so focused on, so taken over by, so obsessed with counting calories and weighing food, and you never feel as though you do enough exercise, you keep missing out on your life.

The process — life itself — is the goal, not some number that weighs your self-esteem more than anything else. If you aren't present for your process, your life, you get to where you believe the goal is and you raise the proverbial bar. You make another goal. And then you push to get to that goal. And then you make another one. And in the meantime, you keep missing out on living, on your life. And then you wonder how it all went by so fast and where you were while it was happening. That is how people get to the end of their lives and suddenly realize they missed the gifts; the small moments. The ordinary moments, on the way to the goal, under the elusive spell of "I'll feel better when ..." This moment, right now, is it. How will you take care of you in this moment?

Trade your expectation for appreciation and the world
changes instantly.

Tony Robbins

Hormone Havoc

Sex hormones have a powerful impact on whether body fat is burnt or stored. They can also impact your mood, whether you feel anxious or calm, withdrawn or angry, and hence the food choices you make and the way you speak to yourself and those you love the most in the world. They affect us physically and also emotionally.

It is important to understand how they work in the body, as well as the healthy patterns and ratios of their production. I find when you understand how your body works, change is more compelling and sustained. Rather than you feeling like someone told you to make a change to your refined sugar intake, for example, once you learn how your sex hormones are made and regulated by your body, your impetus to change comes from a different place; one where sustained change is more likely. So here is how sex hormones influence body shape and size, entirely separately from anything the calorie equation considers.

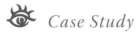 *Case Study*

Amelia's Story

Amelia was a 46-year-old woman who came to see me to lose weight. In our first session, she said she was "completely frustrated" that she had lost no weight since starting her calorie-restricted diet and increasing her exercise, over six months ago. She was very disheartened. Given my approach is predicated on the concept that you have to be healthy to lose weight, I felt there had to more going on for this lovely lady. And indeed there was.

I asked her my zillions of questions, among which are some that explore the menstrual cycle and symptoms the body will present with if sex hormones are too high or too low. Amelia had a regular 28-day menstrual cycle, but she suffered terribly from about day 18 onwards each month. Her weight would increase by 2–3 kilograms around this time, and this would only go once she started menstruating. Her periods were very painful, requiring the use of painkillers, and she passed a lot of clots. The bleeding was heavy for the first two days, and she worried about leaving the house on these days. Her breasts were swollen tender also from about day 18 onwards, she said. Amelia also reported that she found it very hard not to "fly off the handle" at her children and her husband, and when she did she said the situation rarely warranted her reaction. The anger and frustration she felt were present from about day 18 or 20 onwards, and then she said she would cry the day before her period. Every month. She thought this was normal.

I told Amelia that I thought her symptoms were mostly due to too much oestrogen, and, even if her progesterone was levels were adequate, the excess oestrogen would make them seem too low to the body. Amelia was an analytical person and wanted to have some tests done to explore this. She had tests done for all sex hormones except progesterone on day 2 of her cycle, and all sex hormones plus progesterone were tested on day 21, the day when progesterone is supposed to peak.

On day 21, her oestrogen came back with a score of >3000 (the lab we used can't measure it any higher) and her progesterone was 2. That is extreme oestrogen dominance; a scenario which has become common in women of menstruation age.

Instead of focusing on weight loss, I focused on supporting Amelia with her oestrogen metabolism, in particular, and over the course of four months her PMT symptoms completely disappeared (they weren't just less severe — they had gone) and she went down two dress sizes. Her quality of life and health had vastly improved, because we had solved what was interfering with Amelia's body's ability to utilize her body fat as a fuel. Sometimes, to do that a focus on sex hormone balance is required. And that is what this chapter is all about.

Her plan of action involved both dietary change, and nutritional and herbal medicines tailored to meet her individual needs.

Dietary changes
- Real food
- No refined (processed) food
- No dairy foods (due to her prior medical history), caffeine, preservatives, additives, colourings, refined sugars, alcohol
- Regular consumption of cooked vegetables from the *Brassica* family
- Iodine-rich foods, including sea vegetables such as arame, kombu, wakame (added to soups, stews, casseroles)
- Increase of dietary essential fats, as an oil added to smoothies or used as a salad dressing

Supplements
Some of the nutrients were combined into one tablet, but they are listed here separately so you can see what was included.
- Magnesium
- Calcium
- Iron

- Vitamin B complex
- Vitamin C
- A food-based green supplement

Herbal medicine
Herbal medicines are best tailored to the individual. Amelia's tonic included herbs that supported the liver's detoxification of oestrogen, supported healthy progesterone production, addressed fluid retention, supported the adrenal glands and acted as anti-inflammatory agents.

Lifestyle and emotions
- Relaxation through breathing and restorative yoga
- Prioritizing sleep: a minimum 8 hours per night and in bed asleep by 10pm
- Walking for 40 minutes per day, 5 days a week
- Resistance training, 2 days a week
- Exploring her unmet needs and creating a plan to address these

In females, the ovaries are the main source of sex hormone production; however, both the adrenal glands and fat cells make sex hormones, too. For men, the testes make their sex hormones, as well as the adrenals and fat cells. The body also contains tissues that produce hormones themselves, but are not sensitive to hormone levels in our body. The reason some tissues are hormone-sensitive and some are not relates to the presence of receptors for a particular hormone being present on that tissue. Let me explain.

Hormones and Receptors: Like Locks and Keys

Just because your body makes a certain hormone, that doesn't mean you get the lovely or the not-so-lovely effects of the hormone. For a hormone to elicit its effects, it has to bind to a receptor. The best way to imagine the way hormones interact with a receptor site is like a lock and a key. When they connect, you get the effects of the hormone. Breast tissue, for example, is highly sensitive to oestrogen and progesterone, the two main female sex hormones, because the breasts contain receptors for both of these hormones.

Sex hormones can be delicious substances that give you energy and vitality, and yet they can also wreak havoc on your life. When it comes to a sense of calm, mental clarity, the ability to be patient and not make mountains out of molehills, fat burning, beautiful skin, as well as fertility, very few substances in our body impact us more than our sex hormones.

The main sex hormones we will cover are oestrogen and progesterone, with a particular focus on their role in body shape, size, fat burning, and calm.

Oestrogen

Oestrogen is a feminine hormone (although men naturally make it in smaller amounts), and it plays numerous important roles in the human body, including ones associated with reproduction, new bone growth, and cardiovascular health. Challenges with oestrogen occur, however, when there is too much of it compared to other hormones, progesterone in particular. Oestrogen can also pose a problem if there is too much of one type of oestrogen compared to other types of oestrogen.

The ovaries of menstruating females make oestrogen, and small amounts are produced by fat cells and the adrenal glands. At menopause, ovarian production of hormones ceases.

From a reproductive perspective, oestrogen's role in the female body is to lay down the lining of the uterus, and it does this between days 1 and 14 of a typical 28-day reproductive cycle, with day 1 of the cycle being the first day of menstruation. The oestrogen lays the lining of the uterus down over these first 14 days to prepare the female body for a conception if it takes place. Oestrogen wants a menstruating female to fall pregnant every single month of her life — whether that is on her agenda or not! Remember, our bodies are completely geared for survival, and perpetuation of the human species is a significant aspect of that survival process.

As a result of the biological imperative to conceive each month, oestrogen ensures there is adequate body fat, as most females do not immediately know when they are pregnant. In the event that the woman is a stick figure without much body fat, it is possible that a brand-new foetus may not survive. To prevent this, oestrogen signals fat to be laid down in typically female areas, giving women a pear-like shape to better serve the childbirth process.

Oestrogen is the hormone that makes female breasts bud at the first signs of puberty, broadens hips, and gives women their curves. It lays down fat on a woman's hips, bottom and thighs, and is typically responsible for making the bottom half of a female body broader than the top half. Oestrogen also, unfortunately, promotes fluid retention when it is in excess, and this alone can be very stressful for a female. Her clothes don't fit her the way she would like them to, and when a woman feels "puffy and swollen" it can have a significant ripple effect on her choices for the rest of the day and night; it can affect the food choices she makes, her intimacy, as well as how she speaks to herself and those she loves the most in the world. This can add another layer of stress to what may feel like an already overwhelming life.

Fluid Retention

I am convinced that many women feel fat when really they are either bloated or retaining fluid. As I said earlier, I never weigh clients and I don't encourage them to weigh themselves. I do this for many reasons, but one is that as hormone levels fluctuate over the month so can the amounts of fluid being retained, until the hormones return to balance. Besides, when you weigh yourself, remember that all you are really weighing is your self-esteem. I have met thousands of women who can gain 3 kilograms in a day — and to say that this messes with their minds is an understatement. If you get on the scales in the morning and weigh 70 kilograms, and by the evening you weigh 73 kilograms, especially if you have eaten well and exercised that day — and even if you *haven't* eaten well or exercised that day — it is easy to feel incredibly disheartened and wonder how on Earth this could possibly happen. Weight can feel like just another thing to worry and panic about, which does little to help with your weight loss, given the stress hormones this will likely lead you to generate!

Remember this: it is not physically possible to gain 3 kilograms of body fat in a single day. The only possible cause is fluid retention. Yet, even though the logical part of the female mind knows this, seeing 3 extra kilos on the scales over the course of just a day, or even a week, will make most women, no matter how reasonable they are, feel anxious, impatient, frustrated and generally lousy. And are you more likely to make good food choices when you feel this way? All of this always feels worse if you have been eating well and exercising and still gaining weight, as then women tend to think that this must mean that they have to find the time to do even more exercise, but they don't know where on Earth that time is going to come from because they are already stretched for time.

There can be numerous factors behind fluid retention, and if it is significant and goes on for too long it is best to see your GP. In a nutshell, though, fluid retention can be driven by poor lymphatic flow, a congested liver from too many liver-loaders, mineral deficiencies and imbalances, and poor progesterone production. From an energy medicine perspective, I also encourage you to think about who or what you may be holding onto that no longer benefits you. Perhaps it is a belief or perception that no longer serves you, and your body is simply trying to wake you up to this and get you to change. So many of us fear change, whether we realize this or not.

Excess oestrogen can be another likely culprit when it comes to fluid retention. It can also drive headaches, including migraines, increase blood clotting, decrease libido, interfere with thyroid hormone production, and, due to its relationship with progesterone, lead us to feel like we have to do everything with haste. These are big health consequences, all because there is too much of one little hormone.

Powerful Progesterone

Progesterone plays a variety of roles in the human body. From a reproductive perspective, its job is to hold in place the lining of the uterus that oestrogen lays down between days 1 and 14 of your cycle. If your body detects that a conception has taken place, the lining of the uterus needs to be maintained and thickened, rather than shed. As a result, progesterone levels begin to rise. If there is no conception, the lining of the uterus is not needed, and progesterone levels fall away, which initiates menstruation. When health is optimal, progesterone peaks on day 21 of cycle and, relatively speaking, is the dominant sex hormone from just after mid-cycle until menstruation.

Biologically, progesterone has numerous other roles. It is a powerful anti-anxiety agent, an antidepressant and a diuretic, and it is essential if you are to access fat reserves to burn for energy. Without the right amounts of progesterone, you will always burn your sugar, which may lead to your body having to break down your muscles for energy rather than accessing and burning fat stores; this, over time, slows your metabolic rate. You may also have a tendency towards an anxious or depressed mood — and if you feel like you have a blessed life and yet you still feel flat, add guilt to that emotional cocktail and a degree of confusion about what is really bothering you. You can see how layer upon layer of physical and emotional stress can form, which is a sure-fire way for women to make too many stress hormones that can also then interfere with fat loss.

It is important to note though, that too much or too little of any hormone can pose a problem. The ratios between the amounts of different hormones can also play a role in symptom presentation.

The Relationship Between Sex and Stress Hormones

The relationship between sex hormones and stress hormones is fascinating and powerful, and critical for people to understand for a healthy metabolic rate. I would estimate that 9 out of 10 women who see me for consultations enjoy positive changes in their body and general well-being when we address this.

Oestrogen is the dominant sex hormone between day 1 and day 14 of the menstrual cycle. For the first half of the menstrual cycle, a relatively small amount of progesterone is made from the adrenal glands. For the sake of this description, let's call the amount two units. Remember, the reproductive role of progesterone is to hold in place the lining of the uterus, with the additional biological functions of it being an anti-anxiety agent, an antidepressant and a diuretic.

However, as you now understand, your adrenal glands are also where you make your stress hormones, namely adrenalin and cortisol. Adrenalin communicates to every cell of your body that your life is being threatened, even though all you may have done is had an argument with your beloved, when he spoke to you harshly because he felt like a failure at the time. Men usually don't behave well when they subconsciously create a meaning of failure from something that has happened, which could come from a question you asked (without any loaded meaning behind it from you), or because he looked at his bank balance earlier that day and it is not where he needs it to be to feel safe or "successful". Women typically behave in a way they, or those around them, don't enjoy so much when they feel rejected, unloved or unappreciated. This does not excuse poor behaviour, but rather offers an explanation to promote understanding. My point is to highlight that both physical (for example, caffeine) and emotional (for example, a perception of pressure or creating a meaning of rejection from an argument) processes can drive adrenalin production and communicate that danger is present.

We now know that when you are internally rattled, cortisol communicates to every cell in your body that there is no food left in the world, and as a result it wants your body to break down muscle and store fat. Even though food is abundant for you, and your cortisol production is likely to be coming from areas of your life about which you feel uncertain, your body relates it to the historical causes of long-term stress and the ensuing threat to the food supply.

Since your body links progesterone to fertility, if your body perceives that your life is under threat and that there is no food left in the world, the last thing it wants is for you to conceive, so it shuts down the adrenal production of progesterone. Oestrogen and cortisol, both signalling fat storage and ongoing stress, remain, while you have lost the counterbalancing hormone that keeps you calm and not anxious, and helps burn fat and get rid of excess fluid. Think about it.

In my opinion, the shift away from good adrenal progesterone production due to the constant production of stress hormones, and the metabolic and biological consequences of this, is one of the biggest challenges facing Western women's health today. I spoke about it in my TEDx talk in February 2014 and it creates a major a-ha moment for women attending my weekend events.

This situation alone is a modern-day, monumental shift in female chemistry, and it can torment a woman's emotional and physical well-being. This shift plays an enormous role in whether you feel vital and alive, or whether you have to drag yourself through each day, and why you might feel a need to do everything with urgency. A female can go from feeling happy, healthy, balanced and energized, with great clarity of mind and an even mood, to having a foggy brain and feeling either overly anxious about things she cannot name, or utterly exhausted, as a result of this shift to constant stress hormone production and the subsequent low level (or absence) of progesterone. Physically, she may feel puffy, heavy, bloated and full of fluid, with a sense that her clothes are getting tighter by the minute no matter what she eats, whether this is actually true or not. And that is just the first half of the cycle!

A menstruating female ovulates around day 14 of her cycle, and numerous hormonal changes occur to drive ovulation. Once the egg has been released from the ovary, a crater remains on the surface of the ovary where the egg popped out. This crater is called the *corpus luteum*, and this is where the bulk of a woman's progesterone is generated. Progesterone is designed to peak on day 21 of a 28-day cycle, at around 25 to 40 units (depending on the laboratory doing the testing). If conception takes place, progesterone levels need to climb to continue to hold the lining of the uterus in place. Once the placenta has formed by week 12 of gestation, progesterone levels climb to around 300 to 400 units. Pregnancy is the time when a woman has the highest level of circulating progesterone, which is why many women glow, especially from the second trimester onwards. Once a woman has birthed the placenta, however, her progesterone level plunges from 350 to zero! Fortunately, birth brings on some other feel-good hormones, such as oxytocin, although they tend to be more short-lived.

Historically, babies were welcomed into extended families and communities. Today, a more common scenario (but not the only scenario) is a hospital birth followed by a new mother at home alone with her newborn during the day while her partner continues to work to pay the mortgage and other bills. If there are challenges in their relationship, or challenges caused by the needs of other children, financial stress, ill or aging parents, an unwell newborn or simply one who won't sleep, the new home environment with baby can be highly stressful. Another common stressful scenario is where a new mother has made what she thought would be a welcome transition (temporarily or permanently) from a corporate career to staying at home with her baby, but is now second-guessing her decision. The guilt and confusion around this scenario can be overwhelming. Such scenarios do not promote the restoration of adrenal progesterone levels, as the body is so busy making stress hormones that it is not "safe" for the new mum to make the fertility-linked progesterone.

Remember, progesterone is one of the most powerful anti-anxiety and antidepressant substances the body makes. On the other hand, if mum and baby do have support, and the new mum doesn't feel she is alone with her new precious bundle — whether this is simply due to the mother's beliefs, attitudes and perceptions, or her actual physical support from other people — then adrenal progesterone levels are far more likely to be restored, and her chemistry is all the better for it.

If conception does not take place during a menstrual cycle, maintaining the lining of the uterus is no longer necessary and progesterone levels fall, allowing a female to bleed. However, something that is common today is *luteal phase insufficiency*, where ovarian progesterone production is poor and the peak of 25 units in the second half of the cycle is not reached. In this situation, progesterone may be the dominant hormone from day 16 to day 18 of the cycle, but it falls away too soon (it is supposed to be dominant from just after mid-cycle until around day 27), and unfortunately oestrogen becomes dominant leading into the menstrual bleed.

This oestrogen dominance is the biochemical basis of premenstrual syndrome (PMS; also known as premenstrual tension, PMT), which causes grief for the woman, and potentially for those around her at times. When PMS occurs, it can be because oestrogen is dominant for all but 2 or 3 days of a 28-day cycle, meaning that progesterone gets very little, if any, time to rule the roost, and a woman misses out on all of its delicious stress-busting and fat-burning qualities.

When Oestrogen is Dominant

Oestrogen dominance may or may not involve low progesterone. You will see how this is possible when we talk about the liver. For now, simply know that the typical symptoms of *low progesterone* include:

❧ premenstrual migraine
❧ PMS-like symptoms (as outlined below under typical symptoms of oestrogen dominance)
❧ irregular or excessively heavy periods
❧ anxiety and nervousness
❧ feeling like you can't get your breath past your heart.

The typical symptoms of *oestrogen dominance* (which usually also involves low progesterone, but not always) include:

❧ irregular periods or excessive vaginal bleeding
❧ bloating/fluid retention
❧ breast swelling and/or tenderness

* decreased libido
* mood swings, most often irritability, easy to anger, and/or depression
* weight gain, especially around the abdomen and hips
* cold hands and feet
* headaches, particularly premenstrually
* tendency to yellow-tinged skin.

All of these symptoms can lead you to feel lousy and like the lights have gone out in your eyes. On top of the internal impacts, the toll that hormonal imbalances can take on your skin can have a significant ripple effect in a woman's life. When your skin is not great, whatever your age, it can be the source of immense frustration and stress. For countless women, balancing their sex hormones is the key to a clear complexion.

The various forms of oestrogen dominance described above are the most common ones I see in menstruating women. The significant excess of oestrogen being made within the female body, combined with increased oestrogen in our environment (in food and chemicals, such as pesticides), appears to be affecting our endocrine (hormonal) systems in life-changing ways. The impact of this flows to the outside of the body and may present to you as a range of challenges, from congested, pimply skin to body fat that won't budge, or a lack of zest for life.

It is essential to discern whether a woman is suffering from symptoms of oestrogen dominance caused by excess oestrogen, or by significantly low progesterone levels. For the latter it would mean that adrenal and/or ovarian production of progesterone is poor. This person may have optimal oestrogen levels, yet they are challenged with their periods due to low progesterone levels. The hormones that signal ovulation to occur are made by the pituitary gland, making optimal progesterone production reliant on good communication between the pituitary and the ovaries.

Another extremely common scenario is one of oestrogen excess. This can be due to excessive environmental exposures, including to plastics and/or pesticides, and, for some, the use of oral contraceptives or hormone replacement therapy. Another significant basis for oestrogen excess is oestrogen recycling as a result of poor oestrogen detoxification by the liver. The liver actually decides whether to excrete or recycle oestrogen, and, since it prioritizes what it needs to detoxify to keep you well and because the body makes oestrogen itself, detoxifying oestrogen is not as high a priority as, for example, the detoxification of alcohol. This is one reason why there can be so much oestrogen being recycled. A woman can have this month's oestrogen circulating, as well as last month's, and even oestrogen from numerous previous months. Even the best progesterone producer cannot balance out or keep up with so much oestrogen.

An additional oestrogen-dominant hormonal picture is a combination of both of the descriptions above, of poor progesterone production and recycled oestrogen. If we took better care of our liver, this would be far less common in the Western world. As I love to say, these things have become common, but they are not normal. Women are not supposed to get PMS. Your period is just supposed to arrive — no extreme mood swings, no pain, no skin outbreaks, no premenstrual migraines — just menstruation. This is something I explore in depth at my weekend events.

Breast Health

The following is an article I wrote for Breast Cancer Awareness Month. The brief I was given was to write about what makes breasts healthy. Some of it repeats information I have included earlier, but I have left it here in totality to remind you of how vitally important these factors are — and because breast cancer is tragically the leading cancer killer among women between the ages of 20 and 59 in high-income countries, the same population affected by PMS.

Healthy Breasts

When it comes to breast health, there is so much we now understand that contributes to the creation and maintenance of healthy breast tissue. Empowering women to take charge of this incredibly important aspect of their health is vital to the future of all women, and education must begin at a young age. Part of the challenge is deciphering fact from fiction or fad, so let's explore what we know creates healthy breasts.

Hormones, Stress and the Liver

Although the hormone oestrogen does some wonderful things for our health, too much of it or too much of a particular type of oestrogen has been linked to some breast cancers. What is important to explore, when it comes to our hormones, is why is oestrogen so much more of a problem now as opposed to a time in the not-so-distant past? Part of the explanation lies in the production of stress hormones, and part of the explanation lies with the excretion of oestrogen following liver detoxification of this substance.

When we are stressed, we make either, or both, of our two dominant stress hormones, namely adrenalin and cortisol. As a result, levels of another sex hormone called progesterone, which has been shown to be protective against breast cancer (except those who are progesterone receptor positive), fall through the floor as the body links progesterone to fertility. If the body believes that your life is in danger and that there is no more food left in the world, the last thing it wants for you is a pregnancy. And so begins part of the problem with oestrogen — it is dominant in comparison to progesterone. This situation may also arise from synthetic forms of oestrogen, such as from the oral contraceptive pill (OCP) or hormone replacement therapy (HRT).

The second scenario to consider involves the excretion pathway of oestrogen out of the body. Once a molecule of oestrogen has done its job for a specific time, it is transported to the liver where it has to be transformed so that it can be excreted. There are two phases to this detoxification process. Over the years, the workload of the liver in its second stage of this cleaning process can get clogged, just like traffic on a motorway. Where once substances flew through the liver at, metaphorically speaking, 100 kilometres per hour, they might now crawl through at 20 kilometres per hour. When this process becomes terribly overloaded from years of too much alcohol, caffeine, refined sugars, trans fats, or the by-products of bowel congestion (a tendency to constipation), the oestrogen will undergo its first stage of change, but there is no room on the phase two highway, so the oestrogen is released by the liver back into the blood stream. Your body is then faced with the new oestrogen it continues to make from your ovaries — if you are still menstruating — and your fat cells, as well as the recycled form. It is this recycled form of oestrogen that has been found to be up to 400 times higher in women with oestrogen-sensitive breast cancer.

> *A*ll of the cruciferous vegetables (*Brassica* family) have potent anti-cancer properties.

Looking after your precious liver is one of the best steps you can take to ensure that your breast tissue remains healthy. Sadly, many women regularly over-consume alcohol, and it is this regular over-consumption that has been undeniably linked to the development of cystic breast tissue and breast cancer. Women need to get real about how much they are drinking. Heart organizations around the world suggest that two standard drinks per day (equivalent of two 100 mL glasses of wine) with two days off each week is acceptable. Cancer research suggests, however, that if you have a family history of breast cancer, there is no safe level of alcohol consumption. That is a massive statement. If alcohol is something you enjoy, don't drink it daily. Save it for special occasions. Sparkling water with fresh lemon or lime can be a great, refreshing alternative.

Caffeine — coffee in particular — has also been found to play a role in the creation of denser, cystic breast tissue. On the other hand, green tea has consistently been shown in numerous studies to be protective against many types of cancers, breast cancer included. Most people are astounded at the changes in their breasts when they take a break from coffee and alcohol. As a woman living in the same world as all of you, a world with plenty of alcohol and caffeine on offer, I challenge you to take a break from these substances no matter how much you love or depend on them. Do it for one week, one little week out of your very long life. Once you've done that, do it for two. Or, better still, omit them for one or two menstrual cycles, and notice how different your breasts feel.

Food and Movement

When it comes to the aspects of our diets that are essential for healthy breast tissue, vegetables and fruits head the list. All of the cruciferous vegetables (*Brassica* family) have potent anti-cancer properties. Broccoli, in particular, contains sulphoraphane, a compound that helps the body begin to eliminate carcinogenic substances from the body in as little as ten days after it is included in the diet on a daily basis. It also keeps oestrogen from binding to and stimulating the growth of breast cancer cells, a vital step in keeping breast tissue healthy. The great news, too, is that sulphoraphane survives cooking. Eat broccoli, ladies!

Eat fruits and vegetables that are rich in beta-carotene. On average, women with breast cancer tend to have lower levels of beta-carotene in their blood, although researchers cannot say whether this is a cause or a result of the disease. A small-scale study in Italy found that beta-carotene given with other, related carotene compounds increased the tumour-free period among women who had already had breast cancer. The safest and most effective way to maintain healthy levels of beta-carotene is to consume five or more servings of dark-green, yellow or orange vegetables and citrus fruits daily. We must eat our vegetables every day. No excuses!

Make an effort to minimize your consumption of fried foods and charcoal-grilled meats. Also, there is significant evidence to suggest that reducing the consumption of animal foods and basing your diet mostly on plant-based foods is incredibly beneficial to breast health and the prevention of breast cancer.

A growing body of literature suggests that insulin resistance is now a contributing factor in numerous cancers. Insulin is a hormone that can behave like a growth factor. It encourages all cells to grow: fat cells, healthy normal cells, and cells that may be precancerous or cancerous. The best way to limit insulin production in the body is to never base a meal purely on carbohydrates or rely on processed foods. The only carbs humans ate up until the very recent past were those from whole food sources such as berries, legumes and root vegetables. The barrage of highly processed foods, rich in refined sugars, starches and artificial ingredients, we are faced with today did not even exist! Limit your intake of these. People also tend to forget that most alcoholic drinks are packed with sugar.

Remember it is what you do every day that will have the most impact on your health, not what you do sometimes. It is not about going without; it is about getting real about what you, as a woman, already know to be true. You know better than anyone when you have too much of a particular substance in your diet ... whether it is alcohol, coffee or sugar. Make the changes you know you need to make now. You will give your breasts a great chance of remaining healthy in the process.

Lastly, move your body. The benefits of regular movement are well documented for many areas of our health, including a reduction in insulin levels and body fat, both of which, in excess, have been linked to unhealthy breast tissue.

Nutrients for Healthy Breasts

Most of us have heard about the importance of iodine for optimal thyroid function and the prevention of goitre. What we hear very little about is how vital iodine is to breast health.

The breasts concentrate iodine as do the ovaries, and studies have shown that the ovaries in an iodine-deficient state can produce a form of oestrogen associated with breast cancer. This has been shown to be reversible once iodine levels are optimal again. Use a salt that contains iodine, add seaweeds to cooking, or take a supplement to make sure you are getting your iodine. Be aware that you can have too much iodine but most people today aren't getting enough.

Also impacting breast health is our dietary intake and ratio of essential fatty acids. These are predominantly found in oily fish, flaxseeds, walnuts and pecans, evening primrose oil, and borage oil. It can be difficult to eat enough of these vital fats on a daily basis, so a good supplement combining at least fish or flax with evening primrose oils can be a great addition to your daily diet. Start with two capsules in the morning and two at night or one to two tablespoons of the liquid oil.

Another mineral that is essential for healthy breast tissue is magnesium and, coupled with selenium, these nutrients have been shown to reduce the incidences of new breast cancers. Green, leafy vegetables are high in magnesium, while Brazil nuts are rich in selenium. Eat them daily, or take a supplement.

Vitamin C is one of the most important nutrients when it comes to so many aspects of our health. The list of wonderful activities vitamin C performs in the body is almost endless. It helps keep the immune system responding appropriately to stimuli, and hastens white blood cell response times.

Vitamin B_6 has also been extensively researched when it comes to breast health. Eggs are a good source, as are bananas and avocados.

Herbs for Healthy Breasts

Two of my favourite herbs work on the adrenal glands. These are *Rhodiola* and the Ginseng family. Both herbs are considered to be adaptogens, which means they help the body adapt to stressors by fine-tuning the stress response. These herbs tend to have a calming effect on the nervous system, which in turn promotes appropriate sex and stress hormone production, rather than extremes.

Other herbs that have been shown to be useful in creating healthy breast tissue are those that promote liver detoxification and bile production from the gallbladder. Bile is essential for the appropriate excretion of any fat-soluble substances from the body, including cholesterol and oestrogen. Useful herbs include St Mary's thistle, Globe artichoke, *Bupleurum* and *Schisandra*.

Minimize Exposure To ...

The final thing you need to know about the creation and maintenance of healthy breast tissue involves what is best kept to a minimum. Minimizing exposure to growth-factor-like substances, including insulin, may be an important aspect of maintaining healthy breast tissue. Dairy products naturally contain growth factors. Cow's milk, for example, is designed to grow a 40-kilogram baby calf into a 900-kilogram beast. The growth factors naturally present in milk and milk products drive this growth. Humans, however, aren't designed to grow at these rates. If milk must be consumed, sheep and goats are smaller animals, so their milks tend to drive slower, smaller growth rates. Alternatively, nut milks contain no growth factors.

There is also a growing and very concerning body of evidence that points at the importance of minimizing our exposure to plastics and pesticides. They disrupt our endocrine systems and can mimic oestrogen. Recent research out of the United States shows that a large percentage of eight-year-old girls have hit puberty, leading to longer oestrogen production over their lifetime. Furthermore, as women choose to have fewer pregnancies or none, this can also lead to relatively more time spent in oestrogen-dominant states. Researchers suggest that poor diet, lack of exercise, high body fat, and exposure to plastics are the likely culprits for the earlier onset of menstruation. We can make a really big difference to our health and our children's health by getting these lifestyle factors on track.

Reproductive System Conditions

There are numerous reproductive system conditions that involve poor progesterone production or oestrogen dominance, and other hormones such as insulin and/or cortisol can also be involved. Due to this, women with these conditions may or may not find body fat loss a challenge. I go into detail about these conditions in *Beauty from the Inside Out*, and so will keep what is below focused on how they impact on the body getting the message to store fat or use it as a fuel.

Endometriosis

Endometriosis is a condition where the cells that were intended to line the uterus migrate elsewhere outside the uterine cavity and adhere. Common sites for adherence are around the fallopian tubes, ovaries, bladder, bowel, pouch of Douglas (the area between the uterus and the bowel), and peritoneum. These cells respond to the hormonal signals communicating with the lining of the uterus and, as with the endometrium (lining of the uterus), the outlying cells thicken and fill with blood. When menstruation occurs, the cells outside the uterus also bleed, and this can be intensely painful and debilitating. Nine out of 10 women with endometriosis also have irritable bowel syndrome (IBS), which can be even more unpredictable during menstruation. Some newer theories about what is behind the condition involve the immune system, and I have no doubt that, as research teaches us more about the causes of it, women with endometriosis will benefit significantly.

Physiological aspects
On a physical level, endometriosis is a condition of significant oestrogen dominance. That is, there is too much oestrogen, particularly in the second half of the cycle, compared to

progesterone. As you now understand, progesterone doesn't just play a role in fertility, but it is also a powerful anti-anxiety agent, an antidepressant and a diuretic. Think about what life is like with very little of a hormone that plays all of these vital roles. Not much fun!

To get these sex hormones balanced for someone with endometriosis, and hence support fat loss if that is needed, the focus needs to be on both the liver and the adrenals. Remember, the liver makes the decision whether we excrete oestrogen or recycle it, and when the liver is too busy dealing with the typical liver-loaders, it tends to recycle the oestrogen. This means that, even for a good progesterone producer, it can be very difficult to have balanced hormones.

To remind you of the adrenal road to oestrogen dominance, it looks like this. For the first half of the menstrual cycle, oestrogen is supposed to be dominant. The adrenal glands are the only place we make progesterone from at this stage, but they also produce our stress hormones, adrenalin and cortisol. No matter what the reason is for your churning out stress hormones, your body will read it as meaning that the world is unsafe or there is not enough food. So because your body links progesterone to fertility, it therefore thinks it is doing you a great big favour by shutting off the adrenal production of progesterone. Remarkably, this doesn't always mean that you will have trouble conceiving, such is the power of the drive for the perpetuation of the species!

Notice that two biochemical scenarios are involved in endometriosis. Breaking the oestrogen dominance cycle is key, and the road to hormonal balance can be quite different for everyone.

The following is a list of tests that can be useful in providing more insight into endometriosis. They certainly don't all need to be done at once, and diagnosis is typically made from a laparoscopy. But a good place to start investigating is with the hormones at the top of the list. They are:

⸙ salivary hormone profile, including E1, E2 and E3 (this looks at three different forms of oestrogen)

- 2 and 16 urinary oestrogen metabolites (oestrogens are metabolized in two ways: the first pathway [2-hydroxyestrone] is protective, while the second pathway [16a-hydroxyestrone] is more potent, and this test identifies which is the dominant pathway — 2 or 16 — for oestrogen metabolism: the ideal ratio between the 2:16 pathways is two-to-one)
- adrenal hormone profile, including cortisol
- CA-125
- serum protein PP14
- 25-OH-D3 and 1,25-OH-D3 (these are two different forms of vitamin D; typically in endometriosis, the 1,25 levels are deficient while the 25-OH levels are in excess — biochemically, this conversion relies on a process called hydroxylation, which can be compromised in women with endometriosis)
- iron studies, B_{12}, folate, and full blood count
- MTHFR (methylenetetrahydrofolate reductase)
- coeliac profile.

Polycystic Ovarian Syndrome

In polycystic ovarian syndrome (PCOS), the eggs in the ovaries ripen on the surface of the ovary but are not released. They harden and form cysts, hence the name of the condition. As you now understand, to obtain the optimal progesterone levels crucial for fat burning, ovulation is essential, since the majority of monthly progesterone is made by the corpus luteum.

Other hormones are also involved in PCOS. The pituitary gland makes luteinizing hormone (LH) and follicle-stimulating hormone (FSH). Just prior to day 14 of a typical cycle, levels of both hormones increase, but in PCOS both of these hormones from the pituitary gland tend to flat-line. Testosterone, the dominant male sex hormone, as well as other androgens, also tend to be higher in women with PCOS.

Physiological aspects

From a hormonal perspective, in PCOS not only do the two pituitary hormones, LH and FSH, tend to flat-line, but the other female sex hormones of progesterone and oestrogen also tend to be out of balance. Progesterone trends low, while oestrogen tends to be high; however, there are also exceptions to this scenario, where oestrogen is low as well (although, for almost all women with PCOS, oestrogen is still dominant over progesterone).

The androgens, of which testosterone is one, tend to be on the high end of normal or elevated out of the normal range, sometimes dramatically so. And so it wᵣ ᵗke this: high androgen levels in the ovary inhibit FSH, ᵢch therefore hinders the development and maturation of eggs (in the ovary). At this stage in development, the "eggs" are called *follicles*.

Dehydroepiandrosterone (DHEA), another steroid hormone, is found to be elevated in 50% of women with PCOS. The elevated DHEA is believed to be due to stimulation by *adrenocorticotropic hormone* (ACTH), which is produced by the pituitary in response to stress. The excess DHEA then converts to androgens via adrenal metabolism, and, in turn, contributes to the typical elevated androgen levels seen in PCOS. In working with women of any age with PCOS, typically we must first address cortisol production, as health and (if necessary) body fat parameters improve faster when what is at the heart of cortisol production is addressed. It is, however, important to note that not all women with PCOS have elevated cortisol. In fact, some have the adrenal fatigue picture described in the "Can Stress Increase Body Fat?" section. PCOS truly is a condition where the whole endocrine system can be involved; therefore, an individually tailored approach to getting the hormones balanced can be a game-changer.

The skin and adipose (fat) tissue add to the complex aetiology of PCOS. Women who develop hirsutism have the presence and activity of androgens in the skin. Interestingly, 70% of women in the United States with PCOS have hirsutism, while only 10–20% of Japanese women do. Researchers believe that this may be due to both genetic and dietary factors, which is a reminder to eat a high-plant diet (like the Japanese).

With PCOS, the key to improvements usually begins with focusing on stress hormone management. Oestrogen dominance may need to be addressed as well, as it is well recognized as a metabolic feature for most women with PCOS; but just as important is addressing what is usually an elevated level of another hormone, called prolactin. About 25% of women with PCOS have *hyperprolactinaemia* (high blood levels of prolactin), which is due to the message the pituitary receives when oestrogen is elevated. High prolactin can then, in turn, contribute to elevated oestrogen. Intervening in some of these vicious cycles can be the key to achieving change for women with PCOS. Elevated insulin and dysglycaemia are other common aspects of PCOS that require attention. Focus on now knowing where to start, and I suggest that this is with addressing cortisol production.

The following is a list of tests that can offer great insight into PCOS:

salivary adrenal stress profile
salivary female hormone panel, including testosterone, androgens, DHEA
blood tests: FSH, LH, prolactin, E2, free androgen index (FAI) testosterone — free and total
glucose tolerance test, fasting insulin, fasting glucose (to determine if insulin resistance is present)
thyroid blood panel: TSH, free T_4, free T_3, thyroid antibodies, spot urinary iodine
blood lipid profile
pelvic ultrasound.

Oral Contraceptive Pill

The oral contraceptive pill (OCP) is successful at preventing pregnancy because it shuts down the ovarian production of hormones, so ovulation cannot occur. The number of women of all ages I meet who have no idea how this powerful medication works astounds me. I am neither pro-Pill nor anti-Pill; I simply want people to make informed choices. I will say it again: the Pill shuts down the ovarian production of hormones, and the body relies entirely on the synthetic version of hormones being supplied by the tablet. Substances in patented medications, such as the Pill, must be at least 10% different from the form the body naturally makes. They are not identical to the form created by the body.

With the ovaries shut down and no progesterone production occurring from there, the adrenal production of progesterone becomes even more important, yet for too many women the adrenal production of progesterone is poor due to constant stress hormone production.

Menopause

At its simplest level, menopause is the cessation of the ovarian production of hormones. But production continues from the adrenal glands and fat cells. However, as explained earlier, many women now make insufficient amounts of progesterone from their adrenals because of chronic stress. In my opinion, this is such a powerful factor in whether a woman breezes through menopause with few or no debilitating symptoms, or whether the heat and the sleeplessness become overwhelming. If you are approaching menopause, I cannot encourage you enough to ensure that your adrenal function is optimal.

> *I*f you are approaching menopause, I cannot encourage you enough to ensure that your adrenal function is optimal.

If you are postmenopausal, focus on adrenal and liver health. Heat from the body can certainly be due to low oestrogen levels, low progesterone levels, and/or liver congestion. If I meet a client who has tried all sorts of natural oestrogen therapies and used herbs that have an oestrogenic action, such as black cohosh, and they are still overwhelmingly hot and suffering debilitating hot flushes, I will tend to suggest treatments that support their liver.

Remember that in traditional circles menopause is a time when wisdom begins to flow constantly. Trust what you already know inside of you when it comes to your health. You innately know better than anyone else what is best for you. Seek guidance from health professionals, but apply what resonates for you.

Hormones as a Barometer

Menstruation and menopause are feminine and very natural processes. In my experience, they offer incredible insight into a woman's general health, as well as a window into her inner world of subconscious thoughts and beliefs. These thoughts and beliefs drive so much of what we do and how we feel. They can be a barometer guiding you to perhaps eat, drink, move, think, breathe, believe or perceive in a new way, and that can be a great gift that helps you obtain the health outcomes you seek, including how able your body is to regularly use body fat as a fuel, distinct from the number of calories you eat and burn.

👁 *Case Study*

Laura's Story

Laura was 29 years old when she consulted me. She presented with PCOS, and said that she found it impossible to lose weight, no matter how much exercise she did or how she ate. She also said she hadn't had her periods for over a year, and this made her anxious about her fertility.

Diagnosis
An initial round of blood tests showed:
- low total cholesterol
- low HDL (good cholesterol)
- low vitamin D
- low urinary iodine
- elevated androgens
- elevated luteinizing hormone (LH)
- elevated prolactin
- elevated fasting glucose
- elevated insulin
- normal iron studies.

Course of action
The plan of action for Laura involved dietary and lifestyle changes, nutritional supplementation, and herbal medicine. Keeping in mind that what works for one person doesn't always work for another, I share this with you to show you how dietary modification and herbal medicine can make a significant difference.

Dietary changes
- Real food
- No refined (processed) food
- No alcohol, caffeine, dairy products, gluten, preservatives, additives, colourings, refined flours and refined sugars

* Increased dietary essential fats
* Fat from real food if she craved sweet food; keeping real food snacks on hand that contain fats and are also just subtly sweet (such as *Real Food Chef* Chocolate Beetroot Mudcake or Brain Balls)
* Increased cinnamon

Supplements

Some of the nutrients were combined into one tablet, but I will list the nutrients separately so you can see what was included.

* Food-based essential fatty acid supplement
* Food-based green drink
* Iodine
* Zinc
* Magnesium
* Activated B complex
* Alpha-lipoic acid
* Vitamin D

Herbal medicine

Herbal medicines are best tailored to the individual. Laura's tonic included:

* hormonal modulating herbs, such as *Paeonia lactiflora* and *Vitex agnus-castus* (the latter also helps lower prolactin), and other herbs
* blood glucose regulating herbs, such as *Gymnema sylvestre* and *Glycyrrhiza glabra* (licorice)

Lifestyle and emotions

* Relaxation through breathing and restorative yoga
* Prioritizing sleep: a minimum of 8 hours per night, and in bed asleep by 10pm
* Walking for 45 minutes, 5 days a week
* Resistance training 2 days per week
* Exploring whose love she craved the most growing up: Who did she have to be for that person? Who could she

never be? This can help her understand what drives some behaviours and beliefs

Outcome

Six weeks later, Laura had a period. It was light, but we were both thrilled that after 14 months her period had returned. She had agreed to stop weighing herself as this was one of her stressors, but she said that all of her clothes were looser, including her favourite jeans. She had had   low-up fasting blood glucose test after four weeks of diet. , ...ange and this was now back in the normal range.

There is always an answer. You just need to know yours and what *your* body wants.

◈ Stress and Sex Hormone Interactions In Short ...

Over the past 16 years I have observed a significant shift in women's health and behaviour, and part of this is generated from the interaction of stress hormones with sex hormones.

Never before in my work had I witnessed so many females in a rush to do everything and be all things to all people. Never before had I seen the extent of reproductive system and sex hormone challenges that I was seeing. Women were wired. Many of them tired, too. Tired yet wired. And this relentless urgency, this perception that there was not enough time, combined with a to-do list whose myriad items were never all crossed off, was having such significant health consequences for women that I had to write about it, which I did in detail in my 2011 book *Rushing Woman's Syndrome*. I didn't want these amazing mothers, sisters, daughters, friends and colleagues to compromise the quality of their lives in order to live up to, and in, this perceived urgency.

Not that long ago in human history, women were given the opportunity to do what had traditionally been their father's jobs, while maintaining what were traditionally their mother's responsibilities. Since then, what has unfolded for too many women is a frantic double-shift, of working day and night, with very little, if any, rest.

We have made more progress in the workplace than we have in the home. Research shows that if a woman and man both work full-time and have one child, she does twice the amount of housework and three times the amount of childcare he does. So essentially, she has three jobs and he has one. It is time for the dawning of a new era for women, which means it has to be for our men as well.

The perceived need to rush, whether a woman displays it on the outside or keeps it under wraps, is changing the face of women's health as we know it — in a detrimental way, from PMS to IBS, from losing our tempers to feeling like we can't cope. And as you now understand, all of these situations can impact the messages our body receives about whether to burn fat or store fat, regardless of how many calories we have consumed or utilized.

On earlier pages, I have described what is scientifically known as *sympathetic nervous system dominance* and the biochemical changes this drives in the body. I want women to understand the significant way stress can impact the chemistry of their body, and the many body systems it can affect, and offer practical solutions to this.

The role of the nervous system

The nervous system plays a significant role in the stress response, and it has a number of parts. The two branches related to this concept are the sympathetic nervous system (SNS), also known as the amped up *fight-or-flight response*, and the parasympathetic nervous system (PNS), the calming *rest, digest, repair and reproduce* arm of the nervous system. The challenge for too many women today is that they live in SNS dominance, and this can play havoc with weight management, food cravings, sleep quality, patience, moods, self-esteem and overall quality of life.

One of the hormones driving this is adrenalin, which communicates to every cell in the body that your life is in danger. As I described in my TEDx talk, science suggests humans have been on the planet for between 100,000 and 150,000 years, and for the entirety of that history that is what adrenalin has meant to the body. The nervous system doesn't know that the adrenalin amping you up is not from a physical threat to your life but rather your body's response to the caffeine you drink and/or your perception of pressure.

When we live on adrenalin we tend not to sleep restoratively, we crave (and give in and eat) sugar despite our best intentions, and we find it harder and harder to utilize stored body fat as a fuel, instead burning glucose. Yet when we primarily burn glucose as a fuel (instead of body fat), because it is our "get out of danger" fuel, the body can't risk the glucose fuel tank getting too low, so the desire for sweet food gets switched on ... Hello, harsh self-talk, when you give in to your sweet cravings even though you said you wouldn't!

Sex hormone imbalances

One of the biggest challenges facing women's health today is the way stress hormone production is interfering with sex hormone balance. Too many women now suffer with premenstrual syndrome (PMS), polycystic ovarian syndrome (PCOS) or endometriosis, and experience debilitating menopauses, which can have both physical and emotional health consequences.

From painful periods to fluid retention, from anxiety to yelling at the people we love the most in the word and berating ourselves afterwards, it has been a long time since women's health has faced such an intense hormonal challenge. This interference of stress hormones with sex hormones is one of the major biochemical factors I want women to understand.

Oestrogen and progesterone are two of a woman's sex (steroid) hormones, and their ratio to one another has the potential to make us happy or sad, vivacious or anxious, clear-skinned or pimply, and our clothes looser or tighter. Big roles for two little hormones!

For the first half of the menstrual cycle, oestrogen is the dominant hormone, laying down the lining of the uterus. Oestrogen wants a menstruating female to get pregnant every month of her life, whether that is on her agenda or not! And oestrogen needs us to have some extra flesh on our bones in case there is a conception, because a woman usually doesn't know when she is first pregnant, and the body's concern is that, if she too thin, she may not be able to supply the growing foetus with the fat, glucose and nutrients it needs to survive.

For the first half of the cycle, we make a small amount of progesterone from our adrenals glands, walnut sized-glands that sit on top of our kidneys. Progesterone's job reproductively is to hold the lining of the uterus in place, yet it performs a host of other biological functions aside from those involved in reproduction.

Progesterone acts as an anti-anxiety agent, an anti-depressant and a diuretic, allowing us to excrete excess fluid. However, our adrenal glands are also where we make our stress hormones; namely, adrenalin and cortisol. As you now know, adrenalin communicates to every cell in your body that your life is in danger, while cortisol says that food is scarce. As your body links progesterone to fertility, the last thing it wants for a woman is to bring a baby into an environment where it perceives she is not safe and where there is no food. The body therefore believes that it is doing you a great big favour by shutting down the adrenal production of progesterone.

Park the fertility aspect of what I have just said and consider the additional biological impacts of this: we make too little of a hormone that helps us not feel anxious, not be in a depressed mood, and allows us to efficiently mobilize fluid. If a woman retains fluid, she usually feels "puffy and swollen", and this discomfort can impact the food choices she makes for the rest of the day, and the way she speaks to the people she loves the most in the world — and intimacy can fly out the window. And that's just the first half of the cycle!

Once ovulation occurs around mid-cycle, the majority of a woman's progesterone is made by the *corpus luteum*, the crater that remains in the surface of the ovary after an egg has been released. On day 21 of the cycle, progesterone is supposed to peak, yet the most common test result I get back from laboratories is "<0.5". In other words, the lab can't find it — can't find the hormone that is designed to help keep us calm, not anxious, not deeply sad and have our clothes continue to fit.

For too many women, oestrogen is dominant (to progesterone) leading into the menstrual period, and this is the typical hormonal imbalance that is the basis of PMS: heavy, clotty, painful periods; swollen, tender breasts; and mood swings that can oscillate from intense irritability to immense sadness, sometimes in the same hour and often for reasons that cannot be identified! This can feel like chaos for a woman ... and for everyone around her.

I like to say that this biochemical and emotional scenario is common but not normal. It doesn't have to be this way. What if the symptoms your body gives you, what if the parts of your body that frustrate or sadden you, are simply messengers asking you to eat, drink, move, think, believe or perceive in a new way? It is time to see them as the gifts that they are. These symptoms can be wake-up calls for women to make changes in their lives that they may not otherwise make, enhancing their health, energy, vitality and greatness in the process.

Why do we do what we do when we know what we know?
So why do we do it? One reason is because we care so much for the people in our lives. On one level this way of living comes from such a beautiful place. It happens because we have beautiful hearts, but, even deeper than that, it happens because we made up a story a really long time ago that we aren't enough the way we are. That we aren't good enough, tall enough, slim enough, pretty enough, brainy enough, on time enough, that we are just not *enough* the way that we are, so we spend our lives trying to please everyone in our realm, putting their needs ahead of our own. We rush around and do all we can to make sure that others love and appreciate us so that we never, ever have to feel rejected, ostracized, unlovable, criticized, yelled at, and like we have let others down.

It is not just the physical health consequences that concern me for women. It is that they live their lives so out of touch with their beautiful hearts, out of touch with how extraordinary they are and in the cloud of false belief that they aren't enough.

It is important to realize that the way we eat, drink, move, think, believe and perceive impacts our need to rush. As a scientist and health professional, I aim to help people live their lives with more PNS activation, because this alone can have the most profound effect on health. From that place, sex hormones are far easier to balance, liver function (ie, detoxification processes) and digestion work closer to optimal, so there is far less bloating, and the thyroid works better, which is also important for the metabolic rate and the ability to burn body fat.

Bring awareness to why you do what you do, and work out what led you there. Awareness, rather than judgment of ourselves, is the first step in this journey to retire from the rush. Please remember that life is precious, that you are precious, and treat yourself accordingly.

The parts of your body that frustrate or sadden you are simply messages asking you to eat, drink, think, move, breathe, believe or perceive in a new way. See them as the gift that they are.

Dr Libby

Driving Metabolic Rate

The calorie equation does not consider thyroid dysfunction or disease in its calculation. Instead, health professionals are taught that an underactive thyroid can lead to a slower metabolic rate, and an overactive thyroid can lead to a faster metabolic rate, although by how much is an estimate and likely to be different for each person.

One of the major challenges with this is the growing number of people with thyroid problems. Some have a fully developed disease — such as hypothyroidism, Hashimoto's thyroiditis, hyperthyroidism or Graves' disease, with the latter two conditions being ones that increase metabolic rate; others, simply a thyroid gland that isn't working optimally, due to nutrient deficiencies, the over-consumption of substances that can interfere with optimal thyroid function, oestrogen dominance or infection. Autoimmune diseases of the thyroid have increased significantly in the recent past, as well.

So let's explore this gland, how it works, how it impacts metabolism, and how to support yours best.

The Thyroid Gland

The thyroid gland is a little butterfly-shaped gland that sits in your throat area. It makes hormones that play an enormous role in your metabolic rate as well as temperature regulation. Every day of my working life, I meet people who exhibit virtually every symptom of an underactive thyroid, yet their blood test results demonstrate that everything is in the "normal" range. (More on "normal" ranges later.)

The production of thyroid hormones involves a cascade of

signals, and glands other than the thyroid are also involved. This means that if there is a problem with thyroid hormone levels, or with debilitating symptoms indicating something with thyroid function is awry, then it is essential to get to the heart of the matter so that treatment can be appropriately targeted.

The thyroid function cascade begins with the *hypothalamus*, a gland that makes a hormone that sends a signal to the *pituitary gland*, a tiny gland that sits at the base of your brain. The pituitary then makes a hormone called *thyroid stimulating hormone* (TSH) that signals the thyroid to make one if its hormones, known simply as T4 (*thyroxine*). T4 is found in the blood in two forms, namely "T4" and "free T4" (FT4). They are the same hormone, except one is "free" to enter tissues while the other is bound up and unable to enter tissues, which is where the work needs to be done. However, T4 and FT4 are inactive hormones, and must be converted into the active thyroid hormone called T3 (*triiodothyronine*). It is T3 that drives your metabolic rate and your capacity to burn body fat. The flowchart below illustrates the hormonal cascade.

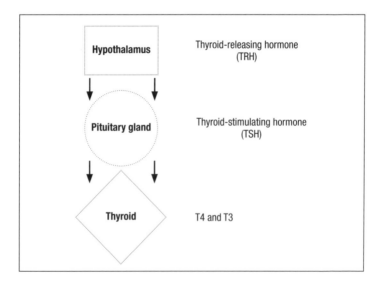

The thyroid hormone cascade: Signalling begins with the hypo-thalamus, followed by the pituitary, which then in turn signals the thyroid gland to make its hormones.

Thyroid Nutrients

There are a number of nutrients essential to the production of optimal levels of thyroid hormones. Iodine and selenium are both vital minerals to this process of conversion, which literally lights up your metabolic rate. Many people today get very little iodine and selenium in their diets, as the majority of soils in the Western world do not contain these essential trace minerals.

Iron is another mineral critical to the creation of healthy thyroid function. Iron deficiency is the most common nutrient deficiency in the world, and this is not OK. There are numerous reasons for this, including: inadequate dietary intake; poor absorption due to (for example) poor gut function; gluten intolerance; coeliac disease; a diet too high in calcium-rich foods, as iron and calcium compete for absorption and calcium wins each time, as it is a bigger molecule; or regular, excessive menstrual blood loss. If someone is iron-deficient, instead of T4 being converted into the active T3 hormone, the T4 gets converted into *reverse T3* (rT3), which is an additional problem for a healthy metabolic rate. To recap: the nutrients needed for healthy thyroid function are iodine, selenium and iron, in particular.

Thyroid Diseases

The thyroid gland can become overactive, known as *hyperthyroidism*, or underactive, known as *hypothyroidism*, and it is the latter scenario which can lead to weight gain that can be difficult to shift until this issue is addressed. Some people swing between an underactive and an overactive situation. The thyroid gland is also susceptible to autoimmune diseases. This is when your immune system, which is supposed to defend you from infection, starts to see the thyroid gland as a foreign particle, like a germ, and attacks it, leading to a change in its function. This can lead to either the overactive picture (with autoimmune involvement, which is known as Graves' disease) or an underactive picture (known as Hashimoto's thyroiditis with autoimmune involvement).

Causes of Poor Thyroid Function

Infection, poor liver function, iodine, selenium and iron deficiencies, calorie intake that is too low for too long, as well as
oestrogen dominance or elevated cortisol are all major factors
that can initiate this process. It is important to work out the
path that leads someone to altered thyroid function, for behind
the "why" lies most of the answer.

Which factors stand out for you? Sometimes many of the
above apply, in which case it is about finding out where to
start.

Hypothyroidism: Underactive Thyroid Gland Function

Because this book is about explaining how our body shape
and size is dependent on more than the calorie equation, I will
stay focused on hypothyroidism (underactive thyroid) and the
whys behind this. So far as an overactive thyroid goes, I will
simply leave it at this: in my experience, stress, specifically the
pace of life and what people demand of their body, is a major factor in
the development of hyperthyroidism. The people I have worked
with who have successfully returned their thyroid function to normal and had a complete remission of
their symptoms have literally changed their life. In all honesty,
they usually change their job, and, if that is not possible, they
completely change their headspace and their attitude to life.
It has been incredibly inspiring to witness this in my clients.

Back to hypothyroidism. The classic symptoms of hypothyroidism are:

gradual weight gain over months for no obvious reason

> *It is important to work out the path that leads someone to altered thyroid function, for behind the "why" lies most of the answer.*

* often feeling cold, sometimes cold in your bones and like you cannot get warm
* tendency to constipation
* tendency to depressed mood, forgetfulness, easily confused
* hair loss or hair drier than previously
* menstrual problems
* difficulty conceiving
* a feeling beyond tired — deep fatigue
* headaches.

Let's explore the roads to an underactive thyroid and where to begin to support your thyroid health.

Infection and poor liver detoxification

A history of glandular fever (Epstein–Barr virus, also known as mononucleosis), for example, is a common road to hypo-thyroidism. Another is liver overload — too many substances and not enough enzymes or nutrients for the liver to deal with the load, particularly in phase 2 detoxification. Treatment of both of these roads involves taking excellent care of the liver, as outlined elsewhere in this book. Additionally, Astragalus is an excellent herb to use for a chronic infection background if an herbalist agrees that this will meet your needs.

Nutrient deficiencies

Eat Brazil nuts daily for selenium. Use Celtic sea salt with iodine and/or cook with seaweeds from clean waters for iodine. Food sources of iron include beef, lamb, eggs, mussels, sardines, lentils, green leafy vegetables, and dates. There is a small amount of iron in many foods, so eating a varied diet is important. Absorption is enhanced with vitamin C. If you do not eat animal foods, do not assume that you are iron-deficient. For some vegetarians, their body utilizes the iron from vegetable sources very efficiently. For others — meat-eaters or vegetarians — they will be deficient, which has dire health consequences not only on thyroid function.

The other option is to take a supplement that covers these

nutrients. There are some excellent thyroid support capsules on the market, so seek out one of these if it appeals, under the guidance of an experienced health professional. Regarding iron, it can be good to have a test before you supplement. Many iron supplements are constipating. Most people find that this does not happen with liquid iron supplements, and there are now some tablets on the market that are highly effective and non-constipating. Zinc and vitamin A are also critical to healthy thyroid function.

Oestrogen dominance

Too much oestrogen suppresses thyroid function, while optimal progesterone levels support its function. Dealing with oestrogen dominance, explained in the "Hormone Havoc" section of this book, is the critical first step if this is the basis for your challenge with your thyroid gland.

Elevated cortisol due to stress

Elevated cortisol as a result of stress decreases the levels of the active, fat-burning thyroid hormone T3, which slows your metabolism. Added to this scenario, high levels of cortisol urge your body to break down muscle to provide glucose for your brain, and the less muscle you have the slower your metabolic rate as well. In the absence of stress, a healthy body converts FT4 into T3, but with elevated cortisol levels, the conversion of FT4 to T3 decreases.

Poor conversion of FT4 to active T3 also occurs if you restrict your food intake. Your body assumes that you must be starving, and therefore it must have a way of slowing down the metabolic rate to preserve those precious fat stores to get you through the perceived famine. It may be frustrating, but your body's primary goal is for survival.

Elevated cortisol also inhibits TSH production from the pituitary. With less TSH, the body produces less FT4. Review what you can do to deal with elevated cortisol, based on the information offered in the "Can Stress Increase Body Fat?" section of this book, if this scenario rings true for you. Poor thyroid function can also lead to elevated cholesterol, and once thyroid function has been treated, the cholesterol returns to normal. I have witnessed this countless times in clients.

Iodine

Iodine is a trace mineral so essential to our health that our body begins to shut down without it. Our thyroid gland loves iodine, and it cannot make thyroid hormones without it. Symptoms of an underactive thyroid were outlined above and if iodine deficiency was involved in the thyroid becoming underactive, increasing dietary iodine intake can make a difference.

Thyroid hormones significantly drive our metabolic rate as adults and our growth as children. Iodine is also essential to the IQ of the developing brain *in utero* and, sadly, studies are now showing that some children in the Western world are suffering from such low iodine levels that their IQ is being detrimentally affected.

Sources of iodine

Soil is a poor source of iodine, and if a nutrient is not in the soil it cannot be in our food. New Zealand, for example, has volcanic soil, which has never contained any iodine, and Australian soils are deficient in iodine, too.

> Thyroid hormones significantly drive our metabolic rate as adults and our growth as children.

While the soil may not be a good source of iodine, the sea is somewhat better. Food sources of iodine include all of the seaweeds, which you can add to soups, stews, casseroles and salads to give them a subtle salty flavour while imparting all of the nutritional value of the minerals. A form of seaweed commonly eaten is nori, used frequently in sushi. Iodine is found in small amounts in some seafood.

Salt was first iodized in 1924; however, iodized salt tended to go out of fashion with the advent of rock salts and Celtic sea salt. Although Celtic sea salt offers the additional benefits of a broad range of trace minerals, it lacks iodine unless it has been fortified. The only concern with conventional iodized salts is that most brands contain anti-caking agents that are potentially not ideal for human health due to some of their ingredients.

The impact of iodine therapy for the maintenance of healthy breast tissue has been widely reported, although it is rarely discussed. The ovaries also concentrate iodine, and studies have shown that a form of oestrogen associated with breast cancer is produced by the ovaries in an iodine-deficient state. This has been shown to be reversible once iodine levels are optimal again.

Substances that can interfere with thyroid function and iodine utilization

There are also substances in food and the environment that can interfere with thyroid function for a variety of reasons. Raw *Brassica* family vegetables, such as broccoli, Brussels sprouts, cauliflower and cabbage, contain substances in their raw state that are known as *goitrogens*. Cooking these vegetables destroys the goitrogens, meaning you still get their valuable oestrogen detoxification properties and other benefits.

Some substances in the diet and environment can interfere with the thyroid's capacity to take up iodine, as any substance that can bind to the same place where iodine is supposed to bind can displace iodine. These substances include fluorine, bromine and chlorine, all of which make their way into processed foods and drinks.

Fluoride displaces iodine. What that means is that, instead of the thyroid gland taking up iodine, if fluoride is present the thyroid will take it up instead. And fluoride doesn't behave the same way as iodine in the body, nor is it able to drive the necessary biochemical reactions for optimal thyroid function. If this happens too regularly for too long, or in too large a dose, thyroid function may be compromised, more so in an iodine-deficient person.

Levels of iodine and supplements

Iodine is a difficult mineral to test for. Accurate tests require you to collect 24 hours of urine, and, remarkably, not all countries offer this testing.

Adult females require 120 micrograms (μg) and males require 150μg of iodine per day to prevent deficiency. It is far more beneficial, however, to individualize doses. Often significantly larger amounts are initially necessary to treat a deficient state, and this can be easily done with one to three drops of a good-quality liquid iodine solution per day, available from some health food shops or which can be made by a compounding pharmacist. It is a trace mineral you can overdose on, though, so it is essential that this be guided by an experienced health professional.

Thyroid Medications

Typically today, if someone has been diagnosed with an underactive thyroid, they are prescribed thyroxine (T4). Some people feel brilliant on this medication and all of their hypo-thyroid symptoms disappear, including their weight gain. If this has not happened for you despite taking this medication, it may be time to try a different approach. After years of taking thyroxine, it will not suddenly start to work if it hasn't yet.

There are numerous brands of thyroxine on the market. If you want to stick with conventional medicine, tell your GP you feel lousy on your current medication and that you would like to try a different drug. I have hundreds of clients who were happily taking one form of thyroxine, and when the thyroid medication that is subsidized was changed to a different brand many of their hypothyroid symptoms returned. Explore this even if your blood levels of TSH, FT4 and T3 are "normal", but you have symptoms.

In my opinion, an excellent option when it comes to hypo-thyroidism is *whole thyroid extract* (WTE). This is taken instead of any synthetic medication and, unlike the synthetics providing only one of the thyroid hormones, WTE provides all of the thyroid hormones. It is essential that you see your GP about this, and, if you so choose, be guided in the transition from a synthetic medication to the WTE, which is made by a compounding pharmacist.

If you have not been diagnosed with a thyroid illness, but you exhibit numerous symptoms, do not rely solely on your blood test results to determine if this is the case. Work with a health professional who will treat the symptoms rather than relying solely on the bloods, and who will monitor both your symptoms and the blood work as you explore treatments. I learnt this in a powerful way with a client whose story melts my heart. I shared this case study in *Accidentally Overweight*, but it is so powerful that I feel it important to bring it to life here as well. See below.

Thyroid Antibodies

The importance of testing thyroid antibodies is best demonstrated with the following case study.

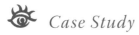

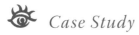 *Case Study*

Patricia's Story

Patricia arrived at my practice for assistance with her health, and when I asked how I could help, she burst into tears and said she knew she has had an underactive thyroid for about 30 years. Her blood tests had always come back as normal, and no one would treat her. She had gained over 100 kilograms in weight over 30 years, and it all began when her dear mum had passed away. Patricia said she ate poorly for about three to four months after her mum passed, but her grief gradually eased and, as it did, she started to eat better again, as she always had. Nothing changed. Her size kept increasing. So then she didn't just eat well, she signed up for a gym membership, and she started to eat even better. Still, her clothes grew tighter.

When I saw her, Patricia was unable to exercise due to knee pain from carrying so much weight (her description, and she thought she was 168 kilograms), but she still ate in a way that did not warrant her size.

Sure, this precious lady had a huge amount of unresolved grief, and, sure, there had been times when she hadn't eaten amazingly. She had, at times, become incredibly frustrated that despite her efforts nothing would shift. But she had also had plenty of years and months of making mammoth efforts with food and movement, with no reward.

Given that Patricia ticked every box for an underactive thyroid, from a symptom perspective, I decided to request fresh blood tests and include thyroid antibodies, specifically anti-thyroid peroxidase and anti-thyroglobulin. Having been taught at university that it was highly unlikely for thyroid antibodies to be elevated and an issue if thyroid hormone levels were in the normal range, I could understand why Patricia's autoantibodies had not been tested, but from a symptoms perspective I could not.

To cut a very long story short, despite her latest thyroid

hormones levels being in the "normal" range, albeit skewed one way (discussed below), Patricia's antibodies were the highest I have ever seen. To put this in context, the "normal" range for both antibodies in this national laboratory is less than 50 (<50). My client's anti-thyroid peroxidase and anti-thyroglobulin levels were both ">6500". Off the scale and through the roof.

When I telephoned her to tell her, she was at first thrilled that all along there had been a reason for how lousy she had felt. Patricia told me later that the anger then surfaced for a life she felt she had missed out on because this was not picked up. She had remained very shy, which she blamed on her size, and on reflection was very sad that she had not met a partner with whom to share her life. She decided to seek out the most natural approach she could for her very underactive thyroid, and, after considerable weight fell off her over the first three months, Patricia booked her first overseas holiday.

There is always a why. You just have to find it.

Blood Tests and "Normal" Ranges

The whole idea of a normal range is necessary, as cut-off points help indicate when something may be abnormal, and it would be chaotic without them. They are a wonderful guide; and I choose the word "guide" with purpose, because for some parameters they are not definitive.

Ranges and What is "Normal"

I have great concerns when we base the future of a person's health on blood tests alone. According to Dr Karen Coates, an insightful and pioneering GP and co-author of *Embracing the Warrior: An essential guide for women*, the normal range for some blood tests is calculated periodically by each pathology laboratory to ensure that the reference range printed on the test results is "accurate". On the morning of this day, the first

100 blood samples received are tested for their (in this case) TSH levels in order to determine the reference range. The same could also be said of iron levels, for example. But why do people usually have blood tests? Because they are feeling particularly spritely that day? No! Most often, the precise opposite is true! Yet, we base our "normal" ranges on these figures.

Furthermore, it is also important to understand how the "average" amount of a particular nutrient or hormone is calculated. Mathematically, the top reference point is calculated to be "two standard deviations" above the average, while the bottom figure is "two standard deviations" below the average. The arbitrary rules of this method dictate that 95% of the 100 blood samples taken must fall into the "normal" range. The statistical definition of standard deviations insists that only four or five results may fall outside this reference range, two samples below and two above.

The three points I want to make are these. First, the reference ranges for some blood parameters are getting broader. I have seen the normal range for TSH broaden from 0.4–4.0 to 0.3–5.0 and then return to 0.4–4.0. As mentioned below, people at either end of this blood range will potentially look and feel completely differently, and they will more than likely exhibit symptoms. If they are symptom-free, no problem; but my concern is that if we base treatment on the blood work alone and leave people to live with their symptoms with their result skewed to one end of the normal range, we are risking, not optimizing, their health.

This brings me to my second point, which is that you can see from the start that this process is flawed given that it is based on unwell individuals. It is more challenging to create optimal health, prevent disease, and maximize quality of life for people when they are being guided with their blood tests to fall into a potentially unhealthy normal range.

Thirdly, often the first time you yourself get a blood test for a particular parameter is when you are unwell. For example, you might not know that when you are optimally healthy your TSH is 1, even though the first time you have it tested, it is 3.

However, as 3 is inside the normal range, you don't get a call-back, because based on "normal" blood ranges your thyroid function is fine. However, in this case, your pituitary gland is having to churn out three times more TSH ᵗᵒ call out to your thyroid gland to get it to make its hormon   hen in the past it only took one unit of TSH to get that outcome.

Your Blood Tests

I urge you to get copies of your own blood tests and look for results being skewed to one end of the normal range. Let's look at this further.

The normal range for TSH where I live is currently 0.4–4.0. Although those numbers may seem small, someone with a TSH of 0.4 feels and looks completely different from someone with a TSH of 4. Additionally, if your results are not actually outside the normal range, you will usually be told (well-meaningly) that there is no problem with your thyroid.

A common picture I see is a TSH of 2.5 or greater screaming out to the thyroid gland to make FT4. FT4 normal levels are 10–20, and usually, for someone with symptoms of hypothyroidism, their FT4 will be 11. This person typically feels exhausted, has trouble naturally using their bowels daily, has dry skin, very low motivation, brain fog, and their clothes are gradually getting tighter. Their thyroid needs support. In this case, once I have taken a diet history to establish poor trace-mineral intake, I will usually start with iodine and selenium, and sometimes iron (once tested), along with adrenal support, a grain-free diet, and a big chat about their beliefs and what their perception is of what life is like for them.

The Third Prong to Holistic Healing

As you have heard me describe, the third prong to my holistic approach to health — after the biochemical and the nutritional — is the emotional. Louise Hay teaches that thyroid problems represent feelings and beliefs around humiliation, and feeling like you never get to do what you want to do (how many mothers does that describe?!?), and subconsciously they ask: "When is it going to be my turn?" She suggests you develop a new thought pattern of "I move beyond old limitations and now allow myself to express freely and creatively." Underneath diagnosed hypothyroidism, Louise Hay suggests, are feelings of hopelessness, a feeling of being stifled, and a sense of giving up. She suggests you develop a new thought pattern of "I create a new life with new rules that totally support me." Apply this concept to your life if it rings true for you. Park it if it does not.

The Whole Picture

I include this information to offer you a whole picture of your thyroid health, from the conventional function of hormones and glands and blood tests, through the nutritional supports that are essential, including iodine, selenium and iron, to the metaphysical — for somewhere among these three approaches lies your answer. Not necessarily in one or the other; I urge you to explore all three.

> *The* thyroid gland plays a powerful role in metabolism.

You can see from this explanation that the thyroid gland plays a powerful role in metabolism, and, with the nutrient deficiencies, stress and hormone imbalances of modern times, this is another reason why the approach to food intake needs to be focused on nutrients, not calories. When people are healthy, their weight falls into place.

◈ Driving Metabolic Rate
In Short ...

The thyroid gland plays a major role in the metabolic rate and temperature control of the body. Its function, however, is controlled from outside the thyroid gland. The hypothalamus in the brain makes *thyroid-releasing hormone* (TRH), and this stimulates the pituitary gland, also in the brain, to make *thyroid-stimulating hormone* (TSH).

The TSH then acts on the thyroid gland to wake it up to make T_4, the inactive thyroid hormone, and this gets converted into T_3, the active thyroid hormone. Much of the conversion of T_4 into T_3 occurs in the liver — yet another reason to take such great care of that amazing organ.

Iodine is an essential component of both T_4 and T_3. A deficiency of iodine prevents the formation and production of thyroid hormones, leading to sub-optimal thyroid function. As Australian and New Zealand soils are deficient in iodine, we do not get sufficient iodine in the food grown in soil. Seafood contains small amounts of iodine.

If someone is iron-deficient, selenium-deficient or stressed, they cannot efficiently convert T_4 into T_3, as some of the T_4 will be converted into reverse T_3 (rT_3), which adversely impacts metabolic rate. rT_3 is thought to be responsible for the brain damage found in iodine-deficient children. For T_4 to be converted into T_3, *selenium* is essential, a trace mineral that is again deficient in Australian and New Zealand soils. This gives you examples of ways nutrient deficiencies can contribute to weight gain, something that the calorie equation does not consider.

Tyrosine is an amino acid (from protein foods) which is needed to make thyroid hormones. When there are regular, high circulating levels of adrenalin, thyroid hormone production can be compromised, as adrenalin is also derived from tyrosine and may compete with the thyroid for this amino acid. Zinc and vitamin A are also critical to healthy thyroid function.

The *Brassica* family of vegetables contains *goitrogens*,

which in large doses can interfere with thyroid function. Cooking destroys the goitrogens, so these vegetables are best consumed cooked if you have a thyroid condition. It is also best to soak nuts and then rinse them for similar reasons.

Some substances in the diet and environment can interfere with the thyroid's capacity to take up iodine, as any substance that can bind to the same place where iodine is supposed to bind can displace iodine. These substances include fluorine, bromine and chlorine, all of which make their way into processed foods and drinks.

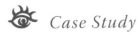 *Case Study*

Mrs B's Story

Mrs B was 34 years old when she presented with what she described as unexplained weight gain and fatigue. I ask a zillion questions, and from that I learnt she also had constipation, dry skin, felt the cold terribly, had dark circles under the eyes, and had irregular periods.

Diagnosis

An initial round of blood tests had found:

* thyroid-stimulating hormone: 6.2 mU/L (high)
* urinary iodine: 38 micrograms/L (low)
* anti-thyroid peroxidase antibodies: 690 units/mL (high)
* anti-thyroglobulin antibodies: negative (healthy)
* ferritin: 12 micrograms/L (low).

Once her results were received, I advised Mrs B to have a thyroid ultrasound via her GP. This was found to be negative for any abnormalities, and Mrs B's GP was happy to monitor her progress, allowing me to treat her (at the patient's request) before re-testing her thyroid parameters to decide if conventional medication was necessary.

Course of action

The plan of action I created for Mrs B involved dietary and lifestyle changes, nutritional supplementation and herbal medicine. Keeping in mind that what works for one person doesn't always work for another, I share this with you to show you how dietary modification and herbal medicine can make a significant difference.

Dietary changes

* Real food
* No refined (processed) food

- No gluten, caffeine, preservatives, additives, colourings or refined sugars
- No goitrogens (all *Brassicas* to be cooked; nuts soaked and rinsed)
- Iodine-rich foods, including sea vegetables such as arame, kombu and wakame (added to soups, stews and casseroles)
- Increased dietary essential fats

Supplements
Some of the nutrients were combined into one tablet, but I will list the nutrients separately so you can see what was included.
- Iodine
- Selenium
- Zinc
- Iron
- Tyrosine
- Vitamin B complex
- Vitamin C

Herbal medicine
Herbal medicines are best tailored to the individual. Mrs B's tonic included:
- *Coleus forskholii,* as it helps to stimulate the thyroid and is a digestive tonic
- *Rehmannia glutinosa,* as it is an adaptogen, helping restore adrenal function (which can be important to address if there has been stress in the lead-up to poor health), and is an anti-inflammatory
- *Hemidesmus indicus,* as it is an immune modulator, which I felt was important given she had thyroid antibodies.

Lifestyle and emotions
- Relaxation through breathing, visualization, qigong
- Prioritizing sleep; a minimum of 8 hours per night, and in bed asleep by 10pm
- Walking for 20 minutes per day every day, until her energy increases and she is able to walk for longer periods

* Exploring where her need to put everyone else before herself comes from, given that she tells others that she does this willingly, however she keeps it to herself that she resents this (she said she feels like she never gets to do what she wants to do)

Outcome

Eight weeks later, Mrs B looked much happier and healthier as she entered my office, and I noticed immediately that the dark circles under her eyes were gone. She reported a significant improvement in her energy, she had had a 30-day menstrual cycle, she was using her bowels daily, and her clothes were looser.

Her re-test results:

* thyroid-stimulating hormone: 3.0 mU/L (normal range; for optimal health, this is still higher than I like it, but is much improved from eight weeks previously)
* urinary iodine: 110 micrograms/L (normal range; much improved)
* anti-thyroid peroxidase antibodies: 380 units/mL (still too high, but on their way down)
* anti-thyroglobulin antibodies: negative (healthy)
* ferritin: 29 micrograms/L (considered normal range, but still too low for optimal health; however heading in the right direction).

*W*ho you are is your contribution to the world and the world would not be the same without you! The world needs you and wants you to recognize all you contribute just by being who you are.

Dr Libby

Fat Storage, Sugar and Appetite

The calorie equation assumes that all calories, regardless of their source, behave in the same way inside the body. However, is this true? One gram of carbohydrate yields four calories as does one gram of protein. One gram of fat gives you nine calories and one gram of alcohol yields seven calories. Yet because each of these macronutrients are metabolized very differently and each drives the production of different hormones which themselves impact metabolism and the way body fat is utilized and muscle mass created (or not), I believe the food from which the calories come matters more than the calories themselves.

Given that science suggests that humans have been on the planet for about 150,000 years, and that Nature has made it relatively hard for us to obtain sweet food, other than in fruits, the amount of refined sugars and flours in the diet now is a significant change. So let's explore what sugars actually are, given that the word "sugar" is often used colloquially, as well as how carbohydrates are metabolized, so you can witness the cascade of biochemical changes they drive, and appreciate the way this may be impacting body shape size beyond what the calorie equation offers.

Sugars

Before answering the question "What is sugar?", it is vital to clarify the precise definition of the word "sugar", as it is used loosely in the modern vernacular and given a variety of meanings.

Defining "Sugar"

Technically, sugar and starch are carbohydrates, with one of the main differences between them being the size of their structures. The term "sugar" refers to simple sugars, *monosaccharides*, such as glucose and fructose, as well as *disaccharides*, such as sucrose, lactose and maltose, which are two monosaccharides linked together. Starches are *polysaccharides* made up of long chains of monosaccharides. Starches are broken down into sugars during digestion.

The simplest way to understand the language used to describe carbohydrates is to think of the "saccharide" part of the words above to mean "sugar" and "mono" meaning "one", "di" meaning "two" and poly meaning "many". All carbohydrates are broken down to glucose during digestion.

Metabolizing Sugars

When it comes to understanding how sugars are metabolized, it is important to understand the action of *insulin*, a hormone made by the pancreas. Insulin is a type of growth hormone, hence its capacity to drive fat storage.

We make insulin when we eat. Carbohydrates elicit the largest production, while protein drives a small amount of insulin release, which is usually offset by another hormone that protein elicits, called *glucagon*, which acts in the opposite way to insulin. People have become confused about and fearful of carbs, and yet we must consume some carbohydrates, as they are vital to the function of our brain, kidneys and red blood cells.

When you consume carbohydrates, whether they are starchy or sweet carbs, they are broken down into glucose. Typical sources of carbohydrates in the modern diet include bread, pasta, rice, all types of potatoes and the other starchy vegetables (including pumpkin and corn), fruit, dairy products, lollies/sweets, cakes, biscuits, pastries, honey, maple syrup and sugar. I guide people to consume carbohydrates from real food, whole food sources.

Influence of diet fashions

I have found it fascinating to ask audiences to shout out sources of carbohydrates. Today, the only carbs audiences tend to identify are the starches ("bread" and "potato" are the first two words out of their mouths every time), which I believe is the result of the high-protein diet era. Eleven years ago, when I asked audiences to name sources of carbs, the first and almost only word out of their mouths was "sugar".

Back then, fat was still the "enemy" of the public health nutrition messages, and the public believed that, so long as there was very little fat in a food, then it had to be good. Bread and pasta are high in what were known as complex carbohydrates and very low in fat, and people ate them by the bucket-load. Back then, there was still some wariness about sugar, as it had been hailed as an enemy in the late 1970s on the back end of the previous high-protein diet age.

You see, nutrition information moves in cycles, and it will continue to do so. To avoid getting caught in the latest fad, I remind you that with food Nature gets it right, and it is human intervention that makes food less nourishing and sustaining for us. My point here is that starch-based foods are carbs, as well as absolutely anything that tastes sweet, unless artificial sweeteners (about which, see comments below) or stevia, a sweet leaf, have been used.

Conversion to, and storage of, glycogen

Glucose from the carbohydrates ends up in your blood stream, and your body identifies that blood sugar levels have been elevated. Your body does not like it when blood glucose levels go high, as too much sugar in the blood can damage the lining of the blood vessels, in a similar way to a free radical. To protect the blood vessels from being damaged, the pancreas secretes insulin into the blood. It is the job of insulin to remove the glucose from the blood so that *homeostasis* (balance) returns to the blood. The health of, and constituents in, the blood must be maintained at all costs.

Insulin first takes the sugar to the muscles and the liver, where it is stored as glycogen, places from which it can be released easily if we need a fast source of energy if we have not eaten for a while. But the size of our muscles is finite, meaning they have their storage limit. Once they are full of glycogen, if more sugar from the blood needs to be removed, then insulin will transport it to guess where? The fat cells. Fat cells have an infinite capacity to expand.

Muscle mass and tone

An essential point to make here is that our *muscle mass* is critical. Do not lose muscle from this point forward in your life. Most favourably, increase your muscle mass. At the very least, maintain it where it is today. Given the glycogen storage capacity of muscles and the ready source of energy they offer, coupled with the metabolism driving power and strength of muscles, I cannot encourage you enough to grow them! You do not need to become a body builder. You do not need to lift huge amounts of weight. Commit to regular resistance training.

Also focus on strengthening the muscles housed in your core. Of course you can also work on the pretty ones that everyone can see, but make sure your core gets attention. Think about this. All of your organs that keep you alive, other than your brain, are housed inside your torso. These organs are held in place by muscles. Over time, due to gravity and poor lifestyle choices, these muscles want to go south, and when this happens they no longer work as efficiently as they once did. Pilates, yoga and qigong are all excellent for core strength, and you can even activate your core while walking or driving sometimes for a little extra bonus.

Food and Insulin

Exploring human food history helps guide us with what to eat, especially when it comes to managing insulin levels. The only carbohydrates humans once ate were legumes, pulses and berries. These days, there are over 3000 snack-food items alone on the shelves of the average supermarket, and this number is growing constantly. None of these packaged foods are what I call *low human intervention* (low HI) foods. Even white bread looks nothing like the ear of wheat from which it came. If you showed a four-year-old an ear of wheat and a piece of white bread, do you think that four-year-old could tell you that the wheat made the white bread? Unlikely, as they are not even the same colour. That wheat has been bleached, rolled and pummelled to create that piece of white bread, so much so that all of the nutrition that was present in the original ear of wheat has been removed, and for that slice of white bread to have any goodness at all the nutrients have to be added back synthetically. And just as an aside, how did you make glue when you were at school? With flour and water. Now, they package it up and sell it to us.

> Remember, it is what you do every day that has the greatest impact.

I am not saying don't ever eat white bread — although many people will feel much better without it. If you love it, buy it fresh from a good-quality baker who uses no preservatives, perhaps on a Saturday morning, or better still buy it fortnightly or monthly and enjoy it. Remember, it is what you do every day that has the greatest impact on your health, not what you do sometimes. If you love it, eat it. Just not truck-loads and not every day. If gluten is a problem for you, of course the white bread has to go completely.

It is big surges of insulin on and off over the day, or constantly high circulating insulin, that are problems when it comes to fat burning and the utilization of calories. If you have spent months committed to exercising and eating well with little or no reward, have your *blood glucose level* (BGL) as well as your *blood insulin level* tested. I have had clients with perfect BGLs, but their bodies are making huge amounts of insulin to keep their blood glucose inside the normal range, and you never know this until you test the insulin. No matter how much you exercise or how seemingly amazingly you eat, you will not access your fat stores to burn in this biochemical state. Insulin must be addressed.

Typical Pattern of Food Intake and Its Consequences

The following is a typical pattern of food intake that I witness regularly. You get up in the morning, inhale some sort of processed breakfast cereal, and race out the door to work. Your blood sugar soars, and your pancreas subsequently releases a surge of insulin. Welcome to fat-storage situation number one of your day. You take shallow breaths all morning due to the perceived pressures in your day. After your peak in blood sugar from your cereal, by mid-morning your blood sugar plummets, and concentration levels are waning.

Looking at your watch, you are relieved to see it is 10.30am. While you have not achieved an awful lot up until now in your day, other than trying to get on top of emails that you actually never seem to get on top of, at least 10.30am means morning tea time, an opportunity to get away from your desk, either with colleagues or by yourself, and head to the nearest coffee cart or café.

You justify your desire for, and subsequent purchase of, a muffin, along with your large double-shot skinny-milk latte, by telling yourself that you have a big day ahead and you will probably go to the gym later anyway. Welcome to fat-storage situation number two of your day, thanks to your coffee and muffin. You return to your desk and push on with some work, but, after about one and a half to two hours, you are fidgety again and want lunch. Your blood sugar has come down from its high, brought on by your mid-morning snack. You look at your watch again — thank goodness it's lunchtime! And out you go for lunch.

You know you feel better in your tummy on days when you don't eat bread for lunch, but you tell yourself that you are busy and you need to be quick. A sandwich, a bagel or a roll is always quick and easy. You inhale it. Then you want something sweet. Hmmm. Chocolate? No, not yet. I'll try a packet of dried fruit first, you think. And, on the inside, your blood sugar and subsequently your insulin levels surge again (fat-storage situation number three for the day). Within half an hour, you feel utterly exhausted, probably bloated, and you are berating yourself because you feel fat. You are, in fact, simply bloated, but your discomfort and the wind building in your tummy, coupled with your protruding abdomen makes you feel lousy. You work in an open-plan office, so you are conscious of hanging onto that wind in case it has an odour. And so the bloating, and hence the size of your tummy, increases over the afternoon.

Headspace, hormones and the roller-coaster

The psychological process that goes on in your head, particularly if you are a woman, after lunch when you reflect on what you have consumed that morning, can be incredibly detrimental to your health. The self-recrimination raises your cortisol levels — that chronic stress hormone which slows the metabolic rate, and can lead to increased body fat — and, hence, expands your waistline. You feel like all you have done is eat all morning and sit on your bottom. You think about the dress you were planning to fit into to wear to an event three weeks from now. Even though all you have done is eat breakfast, a muffin, drink a coffee, have a sandwich, and some dried fruit, in that moment you believe that you will never fit into that dress, and, even though you thought you would go to the gym that evening, having not achieved very much over your morning, you know you will stay back at work and not go. You think about the gym membership that cost you a bomb and that you haven't used for the past three months, and you feel useless. You think again about the "massive" amounts of food you have eaten that day so far, and you berate yourself and your swollen abdomen.

Then — light-bulb! A thought that suddenly makes you feel better flashes into your mind. You suddenly feel back in control. What was that thought? You won't eat afternoon tea! You feel better now, because you have found a way out of your perceived eating frenzy and expanding (bloated) waistline. But your blood sugar and insulin picture over the morning resembled a roller-coaster, and, just because you have decided that you are not going to eat any afternoon tea, how do you expect your blood sugar picture to be any different from how it was in the morning? The answer is that it won't be.

By 3pm or 4pm, your blood sugar has plummeted again, and you feel exhausted. The momentary elation from your "no afternoon tea" thought has vaporized, and you are now "starving" to the point that you could eat your arm off. Your blood sugar is rock-bottom. So, instinctively, what type of food do you think your body will desperately want you to eat in this situation? You guessed it: sugar. Almost nothing raises your blood sugar faster, and your biochemical drive for survival knows it. But you said you wouldn't eat afternoon tea! And now you feel so desperate for it, nothing is going to stand in your way. But if you give in and you eat something, when you said you wouldn't, what emotion do you feel? Guilt. And what stress hormone do you think guilt drives your body to make? Cortisol; hence more fat storage. What a vicious cycle — and one that the calorie equation has no "factor" for. The calorie equation stands half a chance of being closer to the truth if we only ate real food and were robots and felt no emotion.

So you give in and you eat whatever sweet fix you can lay your hands on. Some people will placate the need for food at this time and get another coffee for the day. There is no way a black coffee would hit the spot at this time of day, though. Those who choose the coffee partially feel good because they didn't give in and eat, but then these people know in the back of their mind that an additional coffee at this time of day is not ideal for them either. Over the course of my weekend events, countless women express precisely this to me. But they console themselves with "at least I didn't eat".

Those who do eat feel momentarily better, with yet another elevation in blood sugar and consequently insulin. Hello to another fat-storage situation for the day. And then the self-directed cruel statements silently begin: "You are hopeless. You have no willpower. Look at your stomach." It is the "Will I, won't I? I said I wouldn't, but I did" syndrome!

And, from that headspace, you lament from your desk at 6.30pm — you are still there trying to get on top of the work you didn't do during the day because you were so busy thinking about food and exercise and dresses and your stomach and not passing wind — that you can't go to the gym now because it is already 6.30pm. You still have more work to do, and if you work until 7.15pm, well, there is no food at home and you made a decision to not eat those buy-and-heat meals anymore so you will have to go to the supermarket, and if you go to the supermarket it will then be 8pm before you get home and then you still have to chop the vegetables, and in your mind "that takes ages", and then you still have to cook, eat and clean up, and so it will be at least 11.30pm before you are finished doing all of that, and you probably need to do more work at home that night. But you have to wash your hair in the morning and then straighten it, and so you need to get up earlier to do that ... And then you get up and do it all over again, and you wonder why you can't lose weight when you don't eat "that badly". Hopefully, beginning to understand this cocktail of hormones, which communicate fat storage, is offering some insight into why this may be the case.

Although I may have exaggerated some of the details of the scenario above (or not really!), and written it with very little punctuation to convey a sense of rushing, and also acknowledge there are many variations to what I have described (which may include children, partners, parents or friends), I meet people of all ages who live like this. There may or may not be big, traumatic stresses going on, but there is a daily, relentless juggling act that never ends. It is typical of adults between the ages of 25 and 65, although it tends to be far more prominent in those between the ages of 30 and 55. It comes from a desire to be all things to all people, from being a "pleaser" in your nature, behaviour that was rewarded in childhood. It makes people like you, and you feel good assisting and being there for others, but you never, ever put yourself first. You are exhausted and, if you don't feel that way, you are usually living on adrenalin. It was these scenarios that led me to write *Rushing Woman's Syndrome*.

Hormone cocktail

The cocktail of hormones being made in these scenarios mostly involve cortisol and insulin. In women, this disastrous cocktail in turn interferes with progesterone production, so oestrogen dominance prevails. This down-regulates thyroid function, so you drink coffee or wine, or both, to speed up and cool down, respectively, each day, and your liver gets a regular thumping, and still no one eats enough green vegies. Throw in some emotional confusion and chaos, and you have what is a far too common scenario for too many people. No amount of calorie counting and management will resolve this. Exploring the bigger picture of their lives and focusing on the health of each body system will.

Counting nutrients, not calories

It is time to slow down and make health and the way you nourish yourself a priority, and stop dieting to lose weight. Counting nutrients not calories, eating real food not "food" made in a factory, and a focus on health not weight, will get you to the outcomes you desire. I have witnessed this in thousands of people.

Insulin, Appetite and Fat Storage

What allows over-eating

Please understand that through this entire book I am not suggesting that we are not responsible for how much and what we eat. We are 100% responsible for this. Nor am I saying that willpower plays no role. Of course it does. My concern is that people have viewed food, weight, fat, sugar and size as being as simple as the "calories in versus calories burnt" equation, and that if you eat anything other than what you know to be healthy, then you are useless.

What I want to point out is that hormones are powerful drivers, too, and your drive for safety and survival overrides everything. Regardless of how frustrated you may be with your ever-expanding size — sure you may be eating like a piglet at times and committed to living a healthy lifestyle at other times — take the time to explore your whys. Which hormones might be playing a role for you in this? Do you eat emotionally?

Continuing to rely on an equation that tells you if a food is low-calorie then it is a good choice is redundant. In my opinion, it was a fatal mistake in the first place. A food may be low in in calories but also low in nutrients, and it is nutrients that keep you alive and your biochemistry optimal. And the food may be high in substances your body can't detoxify at a rate necessary for excretion, so you store it in your body fat, further blocking fat burning and loss. The equation doesn't consider that, which, if it did, I would suggest it be called a *toxicity factor*.

Over the past 30 or so years, what has become known as the "obesity epidemic" has unfolded. People tend to judge others and assume that they must eat too much and move very little, and there are times when this is an accurate assessment of why someone is obese. Judgment, however, is worse for you than any chocolate biscuit will ever be, and I want to take this opportunity to remind us all that we have never walked in anyone else's shoes; just as they haven't walked in ours. Bring awareness to when you judge, and take steps to change this reaction to people.

But what I want to explore with you now is what is it about the physiology of the human body that is allowing overweight and obesity to happen? Our biochemistry has what are called built-in negative feedback mechanisms that are supposed to stop us from gaining too much weight. In some people, this does not seem to work efficiently or, if it does, it is biochemically being ignored. Scientists have been exploring what has the ability to block these signals that are supposed to tell our body to eat less and move more, or the signals that tell us to stop eating when we have had enough to meet our physical needs. Clearly, something is getting in the way. And most research indicates that insulin is precisely this block. The entire role of insulin is to store energy, and, in a world of plenty, in a world high in its offerings of processed carbohydrates, through insulin's job of storing energy we gain weight.

As described earlier, insulin moves the glucose out of the blood and into the muscles and fat cells, which results in increases in weight and body fat. But, regardless of size, although this scenario tends to be more distinct in very overweight people, if insulin levels are high, another hormone called *leptin* is supposed to kick in and tell your brain that you have eaten.

Leptin

Leptin is produced by fat in the fat cells, and it circulates through the blood and binds to receptors in the hypothalamus, the area of the brain that controls energy balance. Leptin is supposed to turn off the desire to eat. In addition to this, it also starts to involve the autonomic nervous system (ANS), various parts of which either promote or block fat burning. Through research that suppressed insulin with a drug, it has been shown that insulin interferes with leptin's ability to signal the brain to stop eating. Studies that gave leptin to obese people with the hypothesis that it would shut off appetite have usually found that it is not the miracle pill it was anticipated to be. It appears that insulin stops your brain from being able to "see" leptin, which leaves leptin lousy at down-regulating appetite. The key here is that insulin first must come down for appetite to decrease — especially the desire for carbohydrates — and for weight loss to be sustained.

Exercise and Insulin

Resistance exercise is essential and the best "drug" of all for dealing with insulin. We are crazy if we think exercise only works through burning calories. Twenty minutes of jogging equals one chocolate-chip biscuit. One Big Mac requires three hours of vigorous exercise to "work it off". However, the reasons behind the importance of exercise are far beyond burning calories.

First off, exercise increases the sensitivity of skeletal muscle to insulin. In other words, exercise makes your muscles more insulin-sensitive. Therefore, your pancreas can make less insulin, which leads your levels of insulin to decrease, with the end result of less insulin in your blood to turn glucose into fat. The second reason that movement is important is because, after diaphragmatic breathing (refer to *Rushing Woman's Syndrome* to learn about this powerful mechanism in detail), certain types of exercise are the single best "treatment" to lower adrenalin and cortisol, your stress hormones. More on this in a moment. Cortisol lays down what is known as "bad" visceral fat (cortisol wants your body to lay fat ¹own around the middle so your body will always have ener᷍   urvive the perceived famine), and by reducing it you are decreasing the amount of fat that gets deposited around your middle, and this can also inadvertently reduce your food intake.

Fructose and the Liver: Their Relationship to Insulin

Fructose and Its Sources

The body cannot use fructose as a fuel. It must first be changed into glucose, and an enzyme the liver makes is essential for this. Fructose is the carbohydrate found naturally in foods such as fruits, corn and honey. The trouble, however, is not with the relatively small levels of consumption that people have had for centuries through fruit and honey (unless they have a metabolic or gut-based problematic response to fructose), but rather that human consumption of fructose has significantly escalated over the past 30 years, as it has been added to more and more processed foods. Keep in mind that sucrose (the major sweetener in processed foods in Australia, New Zealand and Canada) is half fructose, and that most processed foods in the United States contain a corn-based refined sweetener such as high-fructose corn syrup, which is also rich in fructose. We were never designed to consume so much fructose.

Over-consumption of Fructose

Unless they are omitting fruit to see if it decreases their bloating or to test for fructose malabsorption or on a low-FODMAP diet, most people can handle two pieces of fruit per day and some honey in tea. There is usually no problem with this except in specific health conditions, mostly due to liver, gut or immune system challenges. Please hear this: it is the *over-consumption of fructose* that is the problem, and potentially the cumulative effects of this on the liver's metabolism that is of dire concern. Fruit, honey and corn themselves are nourishing foods. American statistics suggest that the consumption of fructose has gone from approximately 220 grams a year in 1970 to approximately 25.4 kilograms a year in 2003, an enormous escalation, primarily due to the enormous increase in the consumption of processed foods. Really think about that.

Fructose in processed foods

Originally, fructose was used in food products for people with Type 1 and Type 2 diabetes, and it has what is called *low glycaemic index*, meaning it is digested slowly so it drives a very modest insulin response. Researchers had suggested that fructose was not actually regulated by insulin, and therefore it was presented to the world as the "perfect sugar for people with diabetes". High-fructose corn syrup (HFCS) came on the market after it was invented in 1966, and it began to find its way into American foods in 1975. In 1980, soft-drink companies started to introduce it into soft drinks, and some research suggests that the prevalence of childhood obesity in America can be traced back to this shift. Although, as you now know, the chemistry of fat burning is multi-faceted; widespread use of HFCS certainly hasn't helped, and has added dramatically to the blocks to fat burning.

> *T*he difference with fructose is not the number of calories per gram. The biggest difference is that the only organ in your body that can actually take up fructose is your liver.

Effects of over-consumption

The difference with fructose is not the number of calories per gram. In this respect, it is no different to ordinary table sugar or any other carbohydrate. The biggest difference is that the only organ in your body that can actually take up fructose is your liver. Glucose can be taken up by every organ, and only about 20% of your glucose load arrives at your liver. The fewer loads on the liver, the better! Remember that sucrose (table sugar) is made up of glucose and fructose, so sucrose, too, places an additional load on the liver, particularly due to its fructose content.

The excessive consumption of fructose has been shown to do three not-so-great things within the liver. First, it drives the liver to make *additional uric acid*, the accumulation of which causes gout. It has also been suggested that elevated uric acid is the basis of some forms of high blood pressure. Uric acid inhibits nitric oxide, which is one of the body's natural blood-pressure-lowering agents.

Secondly, excess fructose consumption initiates what is called, in scientific circles, *de novo lipogenesis*, meaning new fat synthesis, which can lead to problems with blood fats and the ratio of cholesterol and triglycerides (free fat) in the blood. And, thirdly, it appears that excessive consumption of fructose can drive *inflammation in the liver*, which appears to stop the insulin receptors in your liver from working effectively. When this happens, insulin levels throughout the entire body rise, so even though we link insulin to blood glucose and the pancreas, as that is where it is made, you can also see how blood sugar dysregulation and/or insulin resistance is related to liver function. I say it again: we must look after our liver! The effects of elevated insulin are actually systemic.

As you now know, when insulin levels rise, this tells every cell of your body to store fat, and high levels can interfere with normal brain metabolism of the insulin signal, which is linked to leptin (as described above). If you put all of this together, elevated insulin not only leads to increased body fat, but also to increased fat in the liver and the liver driving more body fat deposition, as well as increased inflammation. My goodness! What you end up with is a *non-alcoholic fatty liver*, which is now considered to be a disease. When this is going on, your brain can't receive the signal from leptin to stop eating, so you consume more (usually carbohydrates; very few people go back for more broccoli for seconds after dinner). What a vicious cycle! Imagine if you threw in a few alcoholic drinks each week on top of that chemical chaos! And so many people do. It is not surprising so many people feel lousy and find it harder and harder to shift body fat.

The condition known as *alcoholic fatty liver disease* involves the death of functional liver cells due to regular excessive alcohol consumption, and globules of fat replace the active, functioning liver cell. This has dire health consequences. However, as noted above, there is now a new disease known as non-alcoholic fatty liver disease being diagnosed in a broad range of people, including teenagers; teens who haven't consumed alcohol, but whose livers have been engulfed by fat and look similar to those of chronic alcoholics — simply from the amount of processed foods and drinks they have consumed. Really think about that.

In America, soft drinks and many processed foods, such as pretzels, contain high-fructose corn syrup, which is either 42% or 55% fructose. In Australia and New Zealand, soft drinks and most of what I call "birthday party" foods contain sucrose. Sucrose, or table sugar, is 50% fructose (the rest is glucose), so both are of major concern in these enormous doses. Ouch, our livers!

Food choices

Before you panic and go to a dietary extreme — which humans are so good at doing, usually to their long-term detriment — fructose, when combined with fibre, such as naturally occurs in fruit, is far better for us (obviously) than cakes, biscuits and lollies. For example, an average-size orange has 20 calories, 10 of which are fructose, and it is high in fibre. A glass of bottled orange juice has 120 calories. It takes six oranges to make that glass of juice, and it contains zero fibre. Dietary fibre slows the rate of intestinal carbohydrate absorption, which in itself reduces the insulin response.

Do your best to choose foods as you would find them in Nature. Don't be a fruit bat and eat eight pieces a day. Two is perfect or, as I said earlier, zero for a four-week trial to get on top of bloating or a problematic gut bacteria profile, if that is warranted. If you have eliminated fruit and are reintroducing it, bring it back first on an empty stomach to start your day, and see how you tolerate it. Remember, one aspect of exploring your health is about giving you answers to pain, discomfort, or even illness in your body, through which four weeks of dietary changes may give you some insight. It is up to you to decide what you then do with your new information.

The Glycaemic Index and the Glycaemic Load

The *glycaemic index* (GI) is the response of your blood glucose to 50 grams of carbohydrate in that food. It is work that was pioneered at the University of Sydney in Australia, and it changed the face of treatment for type 1 and type 2 diabetes, which are in fact two very different conditions, biochemically. A food can be classed as *low GI*, meaning it makes your blood sugar rise very slowly, causing only a small amount of insulin (the fat-storage hormone) to be secreted. On the other hand, a carbohydrate that is digested quickly leads blood sugar to rise quickly, requiring insulin and hence fat-storage signals to surge.

In my opinion, the GI is a very small part of this picture. I like to talk about choosing foods that are *low HI*: *low human intervention*. Nature knows best. The GI goes no way to considering what else is in the food to make it low GI, and some of those substances may take away from your health.

Furthermore, what is now known as the *glycaemic load* (GL) has come to be shown as a far better guide when it comes to foods, if we need a guide other than Nature, which I am hoping you don't. Take carrots for example. Carrots are very high GI. If you eat 50 grams of carbohydrate in carrots (please note: that does not mean 50 grams total of carrots; it is referring to 50 grams of the carbs in carrots, as they contain other substances such as fibre and water), your blood sugar shoots up very high, hence it is a high-GI food. Fructose, on the other hand, is a low-GI food. Soft drinks in the United State have a GI of 53, which is low, and this is because they are based on high-fructose corn syrup. So if all you considered was the GI, you would say carrots are bad for fat storage, and soft drinks are fine, but of course common sense, Nature and, in this case, science must prevail. Enter the GL.

The GL is the GI times the amount of food you would actually have to eat to ingest the 50 grams of carbohydrate. So with carrots, you would have to eat an entire truck-load to go close to eating 50 grams of carbs from carrots. I have not met anyone who has done that, and I am not suggesting you try! So even though carrots have a high GI, they have a low GL, whereas soft drinks have nothing going for them from a nutritional perspective and have a very high GL, despite having a low GI. Plus, we now understand the impact that excessive fructose has on the liver. We are supposed to eat our carbs with fibre, as this helps make a carb low GL. Nature gets it right. Use common sense. Choose low-HI food.

◆ Fat Storage, Sugar and Appetite In Short ...

Insulin:

- ◆ is secreted by the pancreas in response to rising blood glucose levels (What leads blood glucose to rise? Dietary carbohydrates, caffeine, adrenalin [stress])

- ◆ takes the glucose out of the blood to the muscles and the liver where it is stored as glycogen for fuel for later (muscles are finite; we only have so much muscle tissue, which is why everyone should at minimum maintain their muscle mass where it is now, and preferably build on it); a powerful help to blood glucose management and therefore body fat management is a great muscle mass — not only for how they drive metabolic rate, but also for their carbohydrate storage capacity

- ◆ takes any leftover glucose to the fat cells, which can continue to expand infinitely; this is why it is referred to as a *fat storage hormone*

- ◆ when elevated, sends a message to the body to store fat, not burn it

- ◆ when elevated, stops the body from hearing the appetite-regulating message of leptin, which is one biochemical reason for regular over-eating.

Nothing can dim the light which shines from within.

Maya Angelou

Flexitarian Eating

A concept I would love to introduce you to is what I call having a "flexitarian" approach to eating. I want to guide you to be in touch with what your *body* needs, not what your head tells you you want, or what a rule you created for yourself, possibly years ago, dictates, if this rule no longer serves you or the planet.

A flexible approach enables you to nourish your body with what it needs, when it needs it. For example, there will be days when you feel that a meal that includes rice will nourish you beautifully, whereas there may be other days when you feel that rice won't serve you; you may feel like you will feel tired or bloated after eating it. But if you have a rule that says, for example, carbs after 3pm are bad, then you won't eat rice for dinner, no matter how much your body needs what rice offers.

I find people also define themselves using how they eat as a descriptive: "I'm a vegetarian", for example. And I have met countless people who judge others for how they choose to eat, but judgment does not serve you, your health, the planet, or anyone you meet. Eat in a way that feels right for you, and allow others to do the same.

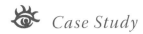 *Case Study*

My story

When I was growing up and during my university education years, it was the low-fat era. So during my university years I avoided fat and followed the dietary pyramid. I also did a lot of cardiovascular exercise. So I could never understand why, when I was doing everything by the book, my weight could fluctuate 1–4 kilograms over a few days when I wasn't doing anything differently from the week before. My diet was low in fat and high in complex carbohydrates such as wholegrain breads and cereals. I lived on breakfast cereal, low-fat milk and fruit, and I have always eaten plenty of vegetables.

Diagnosis

In the 1990s my gut went haywire and I thought I had a bowel disease, the symptoms were so sinister. Blood tests, colonoscopies, endoscopies were all clear, except for what the gastroenterologist said was a "significant infiltration of eosinophils in the lamina propria" of my large bowel. When I asked him what that meant, he replied food allergy or parasite infection. When I asked what I could do about it, he said, "You're the dietician, you work it out." I'm not joking.

This turned out to be one of the greatest gifts of my life, as it set me on a path to think independently. As I said, up until this point I had followed the dietary pyramid and counted calories, and had never understood why my weight would fluctuate for no apparent reason. So here I was faced with debilitating gut symptoms, grateful I did not have a bowel disease, but utterly confused about how to change how I ate, as, based on how I had been educated, I had the healthiest diet on the planet! Plenty of wholegrain breads and cereals, plenty of fruit and vegetables, low-fat dairy products, and small serves of lean meat and fish. I had no history of allergies, and no allergic symptoms, nor did anyone in my family. I was at a loss as to where to start to change my diet.

Course of action

I had started doing my PhD at this stage, and was working with children with autism and their families. For the children, it was often (unfortunately) the foods they craved intensely and ate the most of, such as those containing gluten and casein (a protein in dairy products), which were likely to have the most positive impact on some of their symptoms once they were omitted. If I applied what was at that stage an observation during my PhD, to my own health picture, I looked forward to and ate mostly wholegrain breads and cereals, based on the dietary pyramid. So I decided to omit gluten.

Outcome

After four months of ongoing symptoms, it took only two days for my symptoms to go. Two days. It was a huge relief.

At that stage of my life, the way of eating that nourished me was organic meat and fish, plenty of high-water vegetables, no fruit, nothing at all that was sweet, no onions, no garlic, no coffee, no alcohol, no gluten or dairy products, as my focus was on removing anything that might ferment and therefore irritate the gut lining. I ate mostly soups, stews and casseroles, and I felt incredible. I felt nourished. I ate only real food. I had always eaten mostly real food, but up until this point my diet had contained processed breads and cereals. I had loved them. They were gone. And I couldn't have cared less, because I had my health back and an incredibly powerful first-hand learning experience. And I healed my gut.

Going forward

These days I can eat anything (from a gut perspective). The way I choose to eat, the way of eating that makes me feel great at the moment is still real food, of course, but it is much higher in fat, fat from whole foods. I feel very satisfied and calm with plenty of fat at each meal. I still eat plenty of vegetables, the starchy ones included. I love organic butter. I rarely eat anything sweet: I am not drawn to it, and would rather eat an avocado. I rarely eat cold food, preferring and feeling more nourished by warm, cooked foods.

The way I eat now won't necessarily be the way I eat forever. I actually don't feel like I have a way of eating, other than real food. I eat whatever I feel like. I like to call it being it a flexitarian. I don't enjoy talking about myself, but I decided to share part of my own story with you so you can see that how you eat can change and serve you, depending on other factors in your life. I want to encourage you to be in touch with what your body wants and provide it with the nourishment it needs.

$\mathcal{I}$ have only ever witnessed long-lasting change arise through kindness to yourself, curiosity about what you are doing, and a willingness to act on your own behalf.

Dr Libby

Regular Over-eating

In this section, I am not talking about eating too much when you go to your best friend's house for a dinner party and she has cooked enough food to feed three families. I am talking about when you over-eat every day, when you start eating and you feel like you can't stop. No calorie display, not knowing better, nothing, stops you. It feels compulsive; like you have lost your choice whether you eat too much or not.

Eating in this way has nothing to do with an equation — that is far from your mind if you eat like this. Sure, you will eat more calories than you burn, but knowing that won't lead to behaviourial change. If anything, you will more likely feel guilty, or hopeless, or like a failure, emotions that tend to perpetuate the cycle of over-eating, although most people aren't initially in touch with these emotions as reasons they over-eat.

Regular over-eating is a way we distance ourselves from the way things are when they are not how we want them to be. Really think about that. People (unknowingly) go into survival mode where they (unknowingly) believe "I can't feel this, I won't feel this, it hurts too much, it will kill me", and, when they believe this, they are slipping into what my favourite author Geneen Roth calls "baby skins, old forms, familiar selves".

Young children, especially infants, mediate the pain of loss or abandonment or abuse through the body; there is no difference between physical and emotional pain for them. If the pain is too intense and the defences are too weak, a child will tragically become psychotic and/or die. It is literally lifesaving for a child to develop defences that allow them to leave a situation they can't physically leave by shutting down their feelings or turning to something that soothes them, such as food. But if, as adults, we still believe that pain will kill us, we are seeing through the eyes of the fragile, younger selves we once may have been for a period of time, and relying on the exquisite defence we once developed: escaping. Geneen refers to it as "bolting", and I agree; bolting sums it up perfectly. We bolt. We run. We get out of there. Obsessions of any kind, food included, are a way we leave, because we believe that the pain of staying will kill us.

Accidentally Overweight offers strategies that can lead to long-term, lasting change, as no diet on the planet solves this. No amount of calorie counting resolves the emotional pain that someone uses food to numb. People use all sorts of things to numb their feelings. Food is just one of them. Enquiry and curiosity are the first elements to bring to the table when you want to begin to make a change in why you regularly overeat. Keep in mind that you are eating this way to distance yourself from the perception that things are not how you want them to be, acknowledge this, and find your way to explore this. People often do well with a support person experienced in dealing with the emotional aspects of eating to help guide them with a process like this. It is about getting to the heart of the matter, bringing compassion, and seeing it with new eyes.

Food Is ...

One of the first exercises I do with my clients when they want to get to the heart of why they over-eat (or over-consume alcohol, although we will focus on food here) has nothing to do with how many calories they eat or what they weigh, even though they are seeing me for weight loss. I ask them to complete the following sentence with the first word that flies into their head, no censorship.

I say "Food is ...", and they respond "Yummy", "Delicious", "A pain in the neck", "Life", "Love", "My whole world", "Comfort", "Amazing". These are all words that quickly and easily fly out of people's mouths. For someone who has gained and lost the same 20 or 50 kilograms over the years, food frequently falls into the "pleasure" category. If I am going to guide someone to change the way they eat, and food is their biggest source of pleasure in life, if I don't delve into what else this person finds pleasurable and point this out and encourage them to experience more of this in their lives (such as connecting with the beauty of Nature, their faith, or how playful their puppy is), the food changes will be temporary. Food either needs a new meaning — such as nourishment or energy — or the other pleasure factors need to be amped up in this person's life. Even just being aware of what food means to you is a great first step on the road to lasting change.

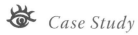 *Case Study*

Julie's Story

One of my favourite examples to share about how this simple process changed a client's after-dinner food frenzy comes from a precious lady for whom food was mostly comfort. Julie had experienced huge emotional trauma, and afterwards food had become her friend, her sweetness, and her joy in life. When she came to see me, she said she was so desperate to lose the weight that she believed had affected her work, as her job was in the public spotlight and she was embarrassed by her growing size. She said she ate entire cheesecakes after dinner regularly and if cheesecake wasn't available, she'd find another cake. This was new behaviour for Julie and had only begun about eight weeks after the trauma. When I did the "Food is ..." exercise with her, it become clear that what she wanted was comfort.

I asked her how else she might find comfort in a way that did not involve food. We had been speaking about how much she treasured her precious daughters, and from her descriptions they sounded very sweet. I felt that when she ate in the evenings what she really wanted was a hug, to be comforted emotionally by another human, or by something bigger (in a spiritual sense), rather than by food. I asked her if she ever stood at the door of her girls' bedrooms and watched them sleeping. Tears immediately sprang to Julie's eyes. As Mark Twain said, "Any emotion if it is sincere, is involuntary", so I immediately knew that this was meaningful to her.

I suggested that, each evening after the girls had gone to bed, Julie complete her usual evening rituals in the kitchen and, instead of going straight to the fridge and into the lounge room for a private sweet feast and the TV, she go to her girls and watch them sleeping. I suggested she notice their breaths, the little lights in their rooms, their innocence, the delicate smell of their hair, and the way their arms poked out from beneath the covers. I invited her to take comfort from their presence in her life. I reminded her that she created them and that, for now, if the only way I could get her to appreciate how truly amazing she was, was by focusing on the little girls she had brought into this world, then that would be the best "medicine" in the world for her. We both cried, and Julie knew with conviction that she had her perfect answer. After just four weeks of practice, weight had fallen off her, and she had not even heard the call of cake after dinner. She had sweetness in spades watching her children sleep.

If all I had done was tell her to stop eating the cake after dinner and taught her to count calories, the pull of the cake would still have been there and, as soon as she felt alone and without comfort, she would have returned to the fridge and had her fill. Then the guilt would have set in, and a feeling of hopelessness that life would never be any different. Instead, by getting to the heart of why Julie ate cake after dinner, she was back in touch with the beauty, comfort and love already present in her life. No calorie equation can account for that.

What Do I Really Want?

When you have eaten and yet you still feel hungry, no food will fill the void for the type of hunger you feel. It is soul food you are looking for at this time, not food food. And the calorie equation goes no way to examining this. It simply makes your hunger "wrong". You feel like your appetite must just be too big, and you worry you will never lose weight, as usually the only strategy people have been given to lose weight is to eat less and move more. So you feel hopeless and like there must be something wrong with you, which only leads you to want to eat more to escape the feelings of your perceived worthlessness that you won't usually even be aware you are feeling.

A powerful strategy to apply in this state is what I have come to call my "What do I really want?" strategy. Create a page in a journal that you divide into four columns with the headings:

What do I want?

What do I really want?

How will having that make me feel?

How else can I feel this emotion in a way that won't harm my health?

First, identify: *What do I want?* Ask yourself and write the answer down. Let's say, your response is "chocolate biscuits". But you have eaten not long ago, and you know you can't be physically hungry, so you ask the next question.

What do I really want? Again, write your answer down. Let's say at first you still say "chocolate biscuits", but you keep asking yourself: what do I really want? And your response might be "a new bathroom", "a hug", "to be thinner", "a boyfriend" or "less financial stress".

But it is not about having those things, as we are governed by how we *feel.* So you ask yourself the next question: *How will having that make me feel?* And your answer might be "happy", "appreciated", "loved", "relieved" or "successful", for example.

Then you follow that up with the final question: *How else can I feel that way that won't harm my health?* And write down your answers. You might say "dance around the house", "read", "watch my children sleep", "phone a friend" or "do something for someone else that makes them feel appreciated", as examples.

> *G*et in touch with what you really want to *feel*, and do the things more often that lead you to feel this way.

Get in touch with what you really want to *feel*, and do the things far more often that lead you to feel this way. Then observe how your desire for food after you have eaten begins to fall away.

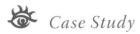 *Case Study*

Mrs P's Story

Mrs P came to see me for an individual consultation, and when I asked how I could help her, and what she wanted to get out of the session, she said she wanted to lose weight. She went on to say that she had heard that I approach weight loss differently from other health professionals, including emotionally, but her issues weren't emotional and she did not want to go there. She told me her problems were all stress-related, and that she just wanted a diet plan. "Give me a plan, I just want a plan. I'm great with a plan, I can follow any plan, just give me a plan and I'll do it," she said.

I am not one to give people plans. I can of course, but it is not how I prefer to work. I want to get to the heart of why someone is overweight in the first place, whether there be biochemical or emotional reasons, or both. This way, they get lasting change and sustained weight loss. Otherwise a plan can feel just like any other diet to a client. However, I am also one to meet people where they are at and meet their needs. So I agreed to provide this lady with a plan of action to meet her nutritional needs under one condition: that if she didn't follow it, she needed to let me know and work out why. She said she would have no problems; she was great with plans.

Four weeks later this lovely — and rather entertaining — lady came back looking a little frazzled. She had not stuck to the plan. And (with kindness) I thought, brilliant! Now we can do the real work that needs to be done.

So I asked what happened, and Mrs P shared that she had followed the plan for three weeks, no problem. And then there was a day when she had dropped her little boy off at the school gate a little late, and there was only one other mum there seeing her child off, too. Mrs P said that she knew this was going to sound embarrassing, but she had always admired this other mum and wished she could meet her and be friends. So she had struck up a conversation with this lady, and they had a lovely chat before she went about the rest of her day.

That afternoon when she returned to pick her little boy up, Mrs P said with intense anger: "The [swear word] looked straight through me. She ignored me. She didn't speak to me. And I was so upset that I forgot about the plan! I ate terribly all afternoon and all night. And I know she didn't speak to me because I'm not in the same league as her. Her son doesn't play with my son. We don't get invited to their parties. Plus I don't wear clothes like hers, and all of the other mothers were around that afternoon, so she would have been too embarrassed to speak to me in front of them. She only spoke to me that morning because no one else was around ..." And she was going to keep giving me reasons why this lady hadn't spoken to her that afternoon, so in the end I stopped her.

I said: "What if I told you that she didn't see you?"

Mrs P replied: "Oh, she saw me alright. She looked straight through me. I should have known. I don't fit in with them, I don't—"

I exclaimed in a louder voice: "She didn't see you! What if that lady's entire focus in the afternoon is to get her child safely across the street and into the car? And maybe she has a zillion things on her to-do list for the afternoon before she gets home to her other children, where she has to bath, feed and put them to bed, because maybe she has a husband who works in a very high-pressured job and doesn't get home until 8.30pm, and after such an intense day he prefers it if the children are in bed and his dinner is ready. And maybe if she doesn't pull all of that off, he yells at her, and maybe then she can't sleep, and will then be exhausted the next day and not be able to be the mother to her children that she wants to be ... It is not about you!"

Diagnosis

Too many adults still live in an emotionally egocentric way. We are supposed to be egocentric as children, not as adults. When you are egocentric, you believe that everything that occurs in your world is because of you. That is what children do. If someone is happy and smiles at them, they link it to something they have done. If someone is upset in their presence, they do the same — think it is because of something they have done.

From such experiences, you create a meaning. You merge the "what happened" (in this case, the lady didn't speak to me) with the story you tell yourself about it (in this case, "I'm not good enough"). And when you scratch the itch of your "not enoughness", you bolt. You escape because you learnt as a child that it was too emotionally painful to stay feeling rejected or ostracized, or unappreciated or unloved, and as a child you didn't have any other resources.

Outcome

I believe that part of being a responsible adult needs to include enquiry into our responses. Once we got to the heart of why Mrs P lived in a cloud of false belief that she isn't enough the way she is, once she saw where that had come from, and also took the wonderful things that had come from what were also painful experiences, then the way she ate and took care of herself completely changed. She didn't need a plan or someone to tell her how to eat. She already knew all of that. Now there was just nothing standing in the way of her belief that she was worth the care she could now show herself.

Unmet Needs

In psychology we are taught that dysfunctional behaviour in children is about unmet needs. I can't tell you how many young girls and boys I have met who have resorted to starving themselves, bingeing, stealing, cutting themselves, lying, bullying, allowing themselves to be victimized, or acting out in some way in a desperate attempt to meet an underlying emotional need.

So if this is true of children, it is likely to be true of adults as well, given that many people live emotionally frozen from some point in the past, in some ways, having not emotionally matured beyond a stressful time in their lives. I hear about it daily. As adults we can function as part of normal society, but behind closed doors where we get triggered — which will show up as an intense emotional reaction to something someone says or to something that occurs — we resort to the behaviour we displayed around the age of the emotional wounding. Much dysfunctional behaviour with food stems from people trying to avoid feeling the emotional pain of the past. Yet they are usually out of touch with the fact that this is what they are doing.

When all we do is try to educate people to change how they eat based on the calorie equation, we negate their feelings further. They can't stick to a "diet" — which will be seen as deprivation, and in some cases starvation, by the person on the receiving end of the instruction — because they have been using food to numb their pain. Plus, no sustained change ever occurs from a place of deprivation and starvation. It always begins with kindness. And I don't use the word "always" in that sentence without careful consideration.

If you take away the mechanism someone has been using to cope for 5 or 50 years, and don't replace it with anything or get to the heart of the base issue and resolve it, they will return to the food or find another way, another obsession or addiction, to numb their pain. When they do this, they feel like a failure, like they are still not good enough, like they are hopeless, pathetic, that they have no willpower. Many people start using food to numb their pain as children or in their teenage years. For some, it is during or after a challenging relationship in adulthood. They have blanketed their feelings so heavily that they can't see that they eat to avoid experiencing emotions they don't want to feel.

When you make food about numbers and strict rules, you set up people who eat emotionally to fail. We have made food solely about education, and sure, people need to be educated. But some of the most overweight people I have met are some of the most educated when it comes to food and nutrition. But it is not a lack of education that leads someone to polish off a packet of chocolate biscuits after dinner; it is biochemical or emotional, or both. And if health professionals fail to address this, the destructive diet mentality that keeps those who struggle with over-eating never feeling that they are good enough, is perpetuated.

I believe that the vast majority of people want to be well. They want to be healthy and feel comfortable in their bodies and have great energy. Let's face it: everything is more difficult when you are exhausted. But most people do not know why they do what they do, even when they know what they know. The emotional needs which food meets — knowingly or unknowingly — for millions of people today, coupled with what I have described as the toxicity factor, the stress factor, the oestrogen factor, the thyroid factor, the insulin factor, the breathing factor, the gut bacteria factor and potentially countless more factors that we are yet to discover, makes simply telling people to eat fewer calories and exercise more redundant, except for those who, for want of a better description, are emotionally not complex. For only without emotion and the aforementioned "factors" is our body shape and size 100% down to the calorie equation.

It is Not About the Weight

It is not about the weight. It has never been about the weight. If a pill is ever discovered that allows people to eat whatever they want and not gain weight, the feelings and situations they turn to food to avoid will still be there. Then they will simply find other ways to numb themselves.

In the film *Groundhog Day*, when the main character Phil, played by Bill Murray, realizes he is not going to gain weight by eating a thousand cherry pies, he eats like there is no tomorrow — because, in the movie, there is no tomorrow. But the buzz dissipates as soon as he realizes he can have as much food as he wants without the usual consequences. When you take the buzz away, all that is left is a "no big deal piece of cherry pie", to quote Geneen. And when you finish the pie, the thing that had nothing to do with the pie, the thing that drove you to eat it in the first place, is still there.

Every time you feel stuck in a time warp, stuck in a recurring pattern of behaviour with food, every time you think you know why you are doing something but you can't seem to make yourself do it differently, have a conversation with yourself. Write down the dialogue with yourself and see what insights it offers. Be open to the outcome, assume nothing, and be ready for anything. Allow it to open doorways into kindness and a new level of self-care. If your relationship with food is a challenge for you, use it as a magical road in to the heart of what it is really about. You are so worth it.

Something to Ponder

What changes for you wh͠ ͠ı change the belief that "life happens ͠u" to "life happens *for* you"?

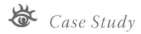 *Case Study*

Mrs M's Story

Mrs M was 52 when she came to see me. She cried within a minute of walking through the door. Over the course of our first session, she shared details of a life having endured much hardship and heartache. She was seeing a psychiatrist once a fortnight to assist with this.

She had come to see me because she was sick of how she ate. She knew she ate emotionally, but couldn't change it. For a period of time Mrs M had lived in the United States, and even with the calorie values printed on menus there, it still had not influenced her choices or led her to make lower-calorie choices. She said it only made her feel more like a failure.

Diagnosis

I don't use the calorie equation in my clinical work. I believe it sets up a poor relationship with food and is inaccurate, in that it does not consider many of the factors that I have discussed in this book, including toxicity, liver congestion, oestrogen dominance, insulin resistance, and elevated stress hormones, just to name a few. But the other significant failing of the calorie equation is how it does not consider people's human needs. This lady clearly over-ate, and she didn't do any exercise at all. In fact she avoided movement. But if all I had done was sit her down and "educate" her about the caloric value of foods, and create an "allowed" list and a "banned" list of foods and drinks, all this would have done was lead her to feel one of the very emotions that prompted her to over-eat in the first place: worthless.

Course of action

Sure, I needed to educate this precious lady about real food and provide her with practical information and recipes to use, but she wouldn't embrace that if she continued to believe she was worthless or unworthy of love or of life. So, as well as the dietary work, we worked on changing the meanings she creates from the interactions she has. When she felt herself wanting to eat when she knew she wasn't hungry, I suggested she identify "what happened" and then identify the "story", the "meaning" she had given to the "what happened". Most of the time, humans merge the two, and the only aspect of the "what happened" that allows it to continue is the story they keep telling themselves about who they must be to have that happen *to them*. What if they changed that to *for them*?

When you get back in touch with how precious life is, with how precious you are, the way you eat changes to a focus on nourishment, not dieting and restriction, and your weight falls into place.

Outcome
Over the course of three and half years, Mrs M lost 62 kilograms. She didn't weigh herself once, she told me, between her starting point of 129 kilograms and the day she decided to see what she weighed, "out of curiosity not judgment", as she put it. That day she was 67 kilograms, but she said she never thinks about it anymore. She has got back in touch with her worth.

The Wrap-up

Sometimes, when people first hear about my work, and they hear me say passionately that it is time to stop dieting, I get feedback that some people initially respond with something like "Oh wow! She's saying not to diet — which means that eating rubbish or bingeing is fine and anything goes!" Yet I am not saying that, as they soon learn.

What deeply concerns me about this is that so many people feel that not dieting means bingeing, or living on poor-quality food. It tells me that people are used to depriving or shaming or punishing themselves as a way of life, and it is that approach to life I am really wanting to challenge. Since how you eat is how you live, deprivation as a way of treating yourself also shows up in how you eat.

For me, the real question I want to encourage you to explore is this: Do you feel the desire, the longing, to live in a different way? To live with ease and spaciousness. To stop punishing yourself or shaming yourself. Not only in your relationship with food, but in your relationship with other people, with work, with money and, most importantly, with yourself. And if you do, that gives you a choice about what to do, how to eat, what you put your attention on, what your priorities are, how you perceive yourself, how you live.

The Three-pronged Holistic Approach to Health

To do this requires a paradigm shift on how you approach what food you eat, and how you eat it. It requires a shift from a focus on weight to a genuine focus on and care for your health.

This means embracing a three-pronged holistic approach to your heath: emotion, nutrition and biochemistry. Let's recap these briefly here in our wrap-up.

Emotion

When you are not hungry, it is not food you want. The food will never be enough, will never fill you, never satisfy you. Rather, it is the associations you have with the food, the stories you tell yourself about the food. It is the memories of that food. It is what you believe that eating that food will give you: a feeling — and it is always a feeling — a feeling of companionship, of belonging, of being welcomed, of no longer being lonely or bored, of being treasured, of deserving the sweet things in life, of being special. When you are not hungry, forget the middleman: food. Go for the treasuring. And start with yourself.

Nutrition

There is no question that humans can over-eat. Certainly it is very easy to do so in today's processed-food-laden world. It is also true they can under-eat. However, the fundamental, underpinning problem is the way we are taught to approach eating: that the only way we can control or influence our body size and weight is via a concept of calories in versus calories burned — based on an equation originating from 1918. This not only ignores the emotional factors that drive food behaviours — which are even more prevalent these days with the epidemic of "not enoughness" I talk about in my TEDx talk — but also ignores the dramatic change in our food supply. Since 1918, there has been a steady and remorseless move away from real food contributing to what I call the "toxicity factor", and an influx of oestrogen-like substances in the environment, which drives fat storage and disrupts our endocrine system.

Biochemistry

Couple this change in food source and content with the advent of the coffee culture, which can drive excess adrenalin production and promotes the fight-or-flight response. Then add to this our perceptions of pressure and urgency mounting daily, as evidenced by stress studies globally, and we have a whole host of factors influencing the metabolic consequences of the calories we eat. Fast-burning fuels are used over slower-burning fat, which is stored to help us survive these "unsafe" times. As this becomes our default setting, our metabolism changes.

The Paradigm Shift

When you base how someone is supposed to eat on a concept that says the only way you can have what you think you want — a slim body, a lean body — is by burning more than you eat, you set people up for a life of obsession and misery. Plus you miss the road to freedom. By freeing yourself from an obsession with food and calories, from intense exercise, and from harsh self-talk, you will find what you seek from the food, but which it can never give you: love.

The healthy alternative is simple:

eat real food
build your muscle mass
get flexible
diaphragmatically breathe
drink mostly water
get eight hours sleep per night.

It is that simple. I always want to write "as often as you can" after these points so that it feels more realistic for you. But the truth is, if I do that, you may not truly appreciate the powerful and wonderful impact a new level of commitment to your health and self-care can bring. I also always want to start points like these with a statement encouraging you to get back in touch with how precious life is, with how precious you are, for when you do that you will treat yourself accordingly. You will do these things without effort. Because that is part of what taking care of yourself looks like.

These points aren't rules. You do not need to follow them 24/7, 365 days a year. You are not required to execute them to perfection. It is what you *consistently* do that impacts your health and your body. This is a way of life; a way of living you return to after a meal with a friend or a holiday. It is how we can support our body in this fast-paced modern world. It is how we can live our best life and make the biggest contribution back. And, along the way, it brings you energy, vitality, grace, freedom and love.

References and Resources

I have included this section for numerous purposes. Firstly, if you enjoy science there are some fascinating publications listed here. These are written in a scientific reference format.

There are also books I've used in the text, listed in full here if further reading in a particular area interests you. The books are listed with their title first.

After reading *The Calorie Fallacy*, you may ask, what's next? I have received and been touched by countless emails from people all over the world saying they feel like I've read their diary when it comes to describing how they feel in the pages of my books. People tell me they want more of this type of information that gives them further insight into their emotional eating patterns. I cannot encourage you enough to check out the array of options on my websites, including my weekend events and online courses. If you relate to the topic *Rushing Woman's Syndrome* but you feel like you don't have time to read the book, you'll likely enjoy the 30-day online *Rushing Woman's Syndrome Quickstart Course* where I guide you on how to retire from being a rushing woman! Take a look at the blog too, at www.drlibby.com.

I also post health information each weekday on Facebook and Twitter. Connect with me there at:

www.facebook.com/DrLibbyLive

www.twitter.com/DrLibbyLive

And on Instagram, find me as "drlibby".

My passion is to educate and inspire, and help people change the relationship they have with their bodies and their health and put the power of choice back in their hands. I don't want food to rule anyone anywhere ever.

It is an honour to assist you in your optimal health journey.

American Psychological Association *Stress in America Report, 2011.* Accessed: www.apa.org 20.07.2014.

Bennett, Jane and Pope, Alexandra. *The Pill: Are You Sure It's For You?* Sydney: Allen & Unwin, 2008.

Cabot, Dr Sandra. *The Liver Cleansing Diet* Camden: WHAS, 1996.

Casey, Dr Lynne. *Stress and Wellbeing in Australia Survey.* The Australian Psychological Society, 2013.

Coates, Dr Karen and Perry, Vincent. *Embracing the Warrior: An Essential Guide for Women.* Burleigh Heads, Arteriol Press, 2007.

Epstein, Donny. *The 12 Stages of Healing.* Amber-Allen Publishers, 1994.

Fasano, Dr Alessio *et al.* (2000) "Zonulin, a newly discovered modulator of intestinal permeability, and its expression in celiac disease," *The Lancet* 355 (9214): 1518–1519.

Gottschall, Elaine. *Breaking the Vicious Cycle: Intestinal Health Through Diet.* Baltimore: Kirkton Press, 1994.

Harris JA, Benedict FG. (1918) 'A biometric study of human basal metabolism' in *Proceedings National Academy Science USA.* 4(12): 370–373.

Harris JA, Benedict FG. *A Biometric Study of Basal Metabolism in Man.* Washington D.C.: Carnegie Institute of Washington, 1919.

Hay, Louise. *You Can Heal Your Life.* Carlsbad: Hay House Inc, 2004.

Hechtman, Leah. *Clinical Naturopathic Medicine.* Sydney: Elsevier, 2014.

Horvath, K., Perman, J.A. (2002), 'Autistic disorder and gastrointestinal disease' in *Current Opinions in Pediatrics* 14 (5): 583–7.

Horvath, K., Perman, J.A. (2002) 'Autism and gastrointestinal symptoms' in *Current Gastroenterology Reports* 4 (3): 251–8.

Horvath, K., Papadimitriou, J.C. Rabsztyn, A., Drachenberg C., Tildon, J.T. (1999), 'Gastrointestinal abnormalities in children with autistic disorders' in *Journal of Pediatrics,* 135 (5): 559–63.

Isganaitis, E. and Lustig, R.H. (2005), 'Fast Food, Central Nervous System Insulin Resistance, and Obesity' in *Arteriosclerosis Thrombosis Vascular Biology,* 25: 2451–2462.

Jin, W., Wang, H., Ji, Y., Hu, Q., Yan, W., Chen, G., Yin, H. (2008), 'Increased intestinal inflammatory response and gut barrier dysfunction in Nrf2-deficient mice after traumatic brain injury' 44 (1): 135–40.

Ley, R.E., Backhed, F., Turnbaugh, P., Lozupone, C.A., Knight, R.D., Gordon, J.I. (2005) 'Obesity alters gut microbial ecology' in

Proceedings National Academy Sciences USA. 102 (31): 11070–11075.

Ley, R.E., Turnbaugh, P.J., Klein, S., Gordon, J.I. (2006), 'Microbial ecology: Human gut microbes associated with obesity' in *Nature,* 444 (7122): 1022–1023 (21 December 2006).

Lustig, R.H. (2006), 'Childhood Obesity: Behavioral aberration or biochemical drive? Reinterpreting the First Law of Thermodynamics' *Nature Clinical Practice, Endocrinology & Metabolism,* Review 2 (8): 447–457.

Lustig, R.H. (2006) 'The "Skinny" on Childhood Obesity: How Our Western environment starves kids' brains' in *Pediatric Annals,* 35 (12): 899–907.

Mills, Simon, and Kerry Bone. *Principles and Practice of Phytotherapy.* London: Churchill Livingstone, 2000.

Müller, B., Merk, S., Bürgi, U., Diem, P. (2001) 'Calculating the basal metabolic rate in severe and morbid obesity'. *Praxis* (Bern 1994) 90 (45): 1955–1963.

Northrup, Dr Christiane. *Women's Bodies Women's Wisdom.* London: Judy Piatkus Ltd, 1998.

Provenzano, Renata. (2006) 'The World According to Karl' in *Fitness Life.* Auckland: Fitness Life; 112–114.

Robbins, Anthony. *Awaken the Giant Within. London:* Simon & Schuster Ltd, 1992.

Roth, Geneen. *Lost and Found: Unexpected Revelations About Food and Money.* New York: Viking Penguin, 2011.

Roza AM, Shizgal HM. (1984) 'The Harris Benedict equation reevaluated: resting energy requirements and the body cell mass'. *American Journal Clinical Nutrition* 40(1): 168–182.

Schofield WN. (1985) 'Predicting basal metabolic rate, new standards and review of previous work'. *Human Nutrition Clinical Nutrition* 39 Suppl 1:5–41.

Shils, Maurice E., Olson, James A., Shike, Moshe. *Modern Nutrition in Health and Disease; Eighth Edition.* Philadelphia: Lea & Febiger, 1994.

Weaver, Dr Libby. *Accidentally Overweight.* Auckland: Little Green Frog Publishing, 2011.

Weaver, Dr Libby. *Rushing Woman's Syndrome.* Auckland: Little Green Frog Publishing, 2012.

Weaver, Dr Libby and Tait, Cynthia. *Dr Libby's Real Food Chef.* Auckland: Little Green Frog Publishing, 2012.

Weaver, Dr Libby. *Beauty from the Inside Out.* Auckland: Little Green Frog Publishing, 2013.

Weaver, Dr Libby and Tait, Cynthia. *Dr Libby's Real Food Kitchen.* Auckland: Little Green Frog Publishing, 2013.

Whitton, Tracy. *Stillness Through Movement.* Gold Coast, Australia: Tracy Whitton, 2011.

CDs
Weaver, Dr Libby. *Restorative Calm.* Auckland: Little Green Frog Publishing, 2012.

Whitton, Tracy. *One With Life.* Gold Coast, Australia: Tracy Whitton, 2011.

My TEDx Talk
The Pace of Modern Life Versus our Cavewoman Biochemistry
https://www.youtube.com/watch?v=tJoSME6Z9rw

Live Events and Online Courses Available at www.drlibby.com
I regularly do speaking tours so check the website for topics, dates and venues. I also run weekend events that offer participants a wonderful restorative experience coupled with in-depth learning of holistic health: the biochemical, the nutritional and the emotional. The *Essential Women's Health Weekend* and the *Beautiful You Weekend* are two favourites that people love.

Weaver, Dr Libby. *Rushing Woman's Syndrome Quickstart Course*

Weaver, Dr Libby. *Condition the Calm Course*

Weaver, Dr Libby. *30 Essential Beauty Gems Course*

Weaver, Dr Libby. *Sensational Sleep Webinar*

Weaver, Dr Libby. *New Year New You Webinar*

Acknowledgements

Thank you to Dr Merv Garrett and my professors from the University of Newcastle in the 1990s who allowed me to be immersed in an environment where critical thinking and questioning what was currently accepted was encouraged and who further fostered my love of human nutrition, biochemistry, immunology, and microbiology.

Thank you to my dedicated team: Jess, Jenny, Dee, Leanne, Sasha, Karen, Aaron and Lisa for all you do each day to make a difference in the world.

Thank you to Kate W. for your contribution to the manuscript, your humour and heart.

Thank you to Kate S. for her genius editing skills and for emails that delight me with the construction of language and the sentiments they convey. I am very grateful to work with you. Thank you to Amy for the layout, your flexibility and the lovely nature-based motifs. Thank you to Stasia for the cover.

Thank you to Joan and her team at Whitcoulls for their encouragement and feedback. We are very grateful.

Thank you to all of the farmers who grow our food and who nurture the soil. Thank you to the growing number of conscious companies who enable people to have access to exceptional quality, non-toxic products. You are all changing the world and I deeply appreciate what you do and contribute.

Thank you to Lorna Jane who inspires me as a human and businesswoman. Thank you for being such an authentic and amazing human and for sharing you with the world.

Thank you to Alexandra for our walks, stimulating conversations and for the joy you bring.

Thank you to Karl for being so clever about the human body

and movement, and for sharing your gold with me. You inspire excellence.

Thank you to my parents for their love, for never quelling my curiosity, for my education, and for having parsley and chickens in the backyard. I am so blessed to have you for my parents and for the friendship that we share today.

Thank you to Chris for helping me share these messages with the world. Thank you for being a visionary, for your insights, your authenticity, and for cracking me up. Thank you for being such a wonderful human, husband, and a super-computer CEO.

And finally, thank you to the incredible people who allowed me to share their stories throughout these pages (I changed their names). Case studies help people learn as they see that others have transformed their health and therefore their body. Thank you to the people I meet at my live events who share their challenges, stories and achievements with me. You inspire me to do what I do.

Meet Dr Libby

Some people have a unique and contagious effervescence about them; an x-factor that compels you to want to be around them; a magnetism that evokes a desire to share in their knowledge; and an energy that, of its own accord, truly inspires and motivates. Dr Libby, PhD is one such person.

Dr Libby Weaver is one of Australasia's leading nutritional biochemists, author and speaker, who lives in New Zealand and Australia. With an extraordinary ability to relate to all demographics, from all walks of life, Dr Libby is a dynamic and highly experienced presenter, who can successfully educate nine people in a boardroom or 9000 people on a stage alongside America's Dr Oz.

She is a five-times number-one best-selling author of the books *Accidentally Overweight, Rushing Woman's Syndrome, Real Food Chef, Beauty from the Inside Out* and *Real Food Kitchen.*

With a background in biochemistry and a natural ability to break down even the most complex of concepts into layman's terms, Dr Libby's health messages are globally relevant, which is why her holistic approach and unique form of education is embraced by audiences across the world.

Her PhD examined biochemical and nutritional factors in children with autism, and her findings have since changed the way the condition is treated in Australia and New Zealand.

Armed with abundant knowledge, scientific research and a true desire to help others get back in touch with how amazing they are, Dr Libby empowers and inspires people to take charge of their health and happiness.

It's no surprise that when it comes to outstanding health, Deborra-lee Furness and Hugh Jackman described her as a "one-stop shop in achieving and maintaining ultimate health and wellbeing".

Real Food Chef

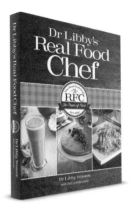

After noticing her clients struggling to come up with ideas for quick and nutritious meals, it seemed a natural progression for Dr Libby to create a series of recipes that have her seal of approval. And so the *Real Food Chef* was born.

The recipes appeal to a broad range of people, from busy mothers to teenage boys. Good, honest food that could be made by anyone; these recipes are sure to impress even the fussiest of eaters and offer nutrient-dense alternatives to your favourite foods. From blueberry cheesecake to satay chicken, *Real Food Chef* is bursting with ideas and images to inspire.

The *Real Food Chef* system focuses on using food in its whole form, including all the food's vitamins and minerals and the natural plant compounds known to support human health; after all, it is nutrients that keep us alive. The recipes are free from refined sugars, dairy products, and gluten, with few exceptions; they are, therefore, suitable for those with some of the more common food allergies, or intolerances. Anyone who wants to optimize their nourishment would benefit from this book.

The *Real Food Chef* concept is a dynamic combination of Dr Libby's nutritional expertise with chef Cynthia Louise's gift for transforming everyday meals into nutrient-dense and incredibly delicious versions of their former selves. As a team, they bring you the why, and the how, to eat real food and amp up the nutrition in your world.

The *Real Food Chef* is a whole cooking system born from a desire to inspire you to eat low human-intervention food, real food the way it comes in Nature. Filled with delicious, nourishing recipes, quotes to inspire, and food education, the *Real Food Chef* is designed to enhance your quality of life and give you more energy to live the life you love.

We eat, on average, 35 times a week and these eating occasions supply the cells of your body with the nutrients to give you optimal health, energy, and vitality. So join this real food journey to discover how real food can revolutionise how you feel.

To help you create these incredible recipes, Dr Libby and chef Cynthia have returned to the *Real Food Chef* kitchen to show you how to make every dish in the *Real Food Chef Video Tutorials*. Chef Cynthia shows you step-by-step how to create your *Real Food Chef* masterpiece and Dr Libby provides the nutritional support, reminding you how each ingredient supports your body, mind, and soul.

To learn more, visit www.drlibby.com

Real Food Kitchen

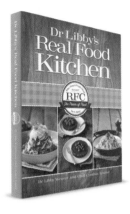

Following on from the phenomenal success of the *Real Food Chef*, the second cookbook in this series takes family favourites and applies the *Real Food Chef* principles to ensure maximum nutrient density of every meal and every mouthful. With 90 recipes covering breakfast, drinks, lunch, dinner, snacks, dressing and desserts — the *Real Food Kitchen* will inspire you to take better care of yourself with the delicious and nutritious recipes featured.

This way of eating has a wide-reaching effect for it is not just about the outstanding nourishment that comes from each recipe, it is also about the what we've left out ... refined and artificial ingredients that have the potential to take away from your health such as refined sugar, white flour and preservatives.

This book provides you with amazing recipes such as Macho Nachos, Coconut Ice, Caramel Slice and Banoffee Pie that serve your health and happiness, and brings it all to life in an easy to use, quick to prepare, and delicious tasting recipe system. Continue your journey to outstanding health, energy, and vitality by embracing the *Real Food Kitchen* way of eating, and witness the transformation as your body, mind and soul responds to true nourishment.

To learn more visit www.drlibby.com

Rushing Woman's Syndrome

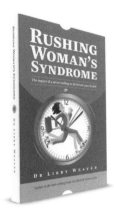

Hot on the heels of Dr Libby's first number-one best-selling book, *Accidentally Overweight*, Dr Libby's second book, *Rushing Woman's Syndrome*, became another number-one bestseller. *Rushing Woman's Syndrome* describes the biochemical and emotional effects of constantly being in a rush, and the health consequences that urgency elicits.

It doesn't seem to matter if a woman has two things to do in her day or 200; she is in a pressing rush to do it all. She is often wound up like a top, running herself ragged in a daily battle to keep up. There is always so much to do, and she rarely feels like she is in control and on top of things. In fact, her deep desire to control even the smaller details of life can leave her feeling out of control, even of her own self.

Rushing Woman's Syndrome examines the nervous system, endocrine system (including sex and stress hormones, the thyroid, and the pituitary gland), and the digestive system, as well as the emotional aspects of why women rush. Dr Libby can simplify even the most difficult biochemistry effortlessly, making this book equally educating and inspiring. What sets Dr Libby's work apart in a world where we are constantly bombarded with health messages, is her ability to search for, and explain, the underlying cause of an ailment, the why. *Rushing Woman's Syndrome* takes you on an emotional journey to help you decipher just where your beliefs are coming from and how those thoughts affect how your body behaves. So come on a journey of food and hormones, thoughts and perceptions, energy, and vitality. It is impossible not to see your life and body from a whole new perspective after reading this book.

Rushing Woman's Syndrome was inspired by Dr Libby's clinical experiences and her empathy for women and the many roles they now juggle. Dr Libby believes we have to be educated and inspired to make changes; her unique conversational style makes you feel like she is speaking right to you. (At the time of writing *RWS*) Dr Libby combines two decades of personal experience, 14 years of university, and 15 years of clinical experience to offer you real solutions to both the biochemistry and the emotional patterns of the rush.

After a multitude of requests for coaching and requests from women who were too busy to read the book (!), Dr Libby created two 30-day video coaching programmes called The Rushing Woman's Syndrome Quick Start Course *and the* Condition the Calm Advanced Course, *which guide you on your journey from rushing back to calm. These courses have achieved phenomenal results with women across the world who are now enjoying life without the rush.*

To learn more visit www.drlibby.com

Accidentally Overweight

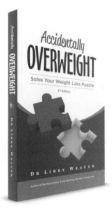

Accidentally Overweight, Dr Libby's first number-one best-selling book, explains what is necessary for the body to be able to access body fat and burn it. So many readers say that *Accidentally Overweight* could easily be called "Optimal Well-being", as the information is relevant to everyone regardless of their health goals.

Whether consciously or subconsciously, many people are frustrated by how they feel about their body, including sometimes its appearance, and this frustration can take up their headspace and influence their moods. Many people eat well and exercise regularly, yet their body fat does not reflect their efforts. This book explains the biochemistry and emotions of weight loss to help free people from their battle with their bodies. It includes strategies to explore emotional eating and specific herbs and nutrients to support optimal biochemistry for the effective utilization of body fat.

What to eat and how much to eat for optimum health and ideal body shape and size can seem like confusing and, at times, overwhelming areas to explore. Right now you could walk into a bookshop and pick up a book that tells you to eat plenty of carbohydrates, as they are essential for energy, and right beside it on the bookshelf will be a book that tells you not to eat carbs because they make you fat and tired.

How on Earth are you supposed to make sense of this well-meaning, but conflicting, information? How do you work out a way of eating that fuels you with great energy all day long while burning fat? What do you do if you feel like you have tried everything to lose weight only to gain it back? Have you ever put your mind to losing weight and made an enormous effort to eat well and exercise regularly for little or no reward? Or perhaps you are actually OK with your weight but you just don't *feel* right? *Accidentally Overweight* answers all of these questions, and more.

To learn more visit www.drlibby.com

Beauty From the Inside Out

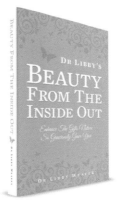

As a society our relationship with beauty is in crisis. We are told that beauty exists only in certain forms, images and at certain ages. We can feel bombarded with images that lead us away from our own unique beauty and encourage us to try to look like someone else rather than accepting more of who we are. While adults can be affected by such messages, these messages can be particularly damaging to children and teenagers who so desperately want to be loved, approved of, considered special and seen as beautiful. There is so much beauty on offer to us 24/7, at any age, inside us, around us, and shining from us. For so many a veil just needs to be lifted so you can experience your own radiance. Let's see what we can do!

When most people think about improving their appearance, they usually focus on a product, another "quick fix". Yet when you consider that the skin cells on your face are a small percentage of the total number of cells in the whole body, it seems crazy that we don't spend more time getting the majority of the cells functioning optimally, leading us to the outcomes we seek.

Through *Beauty From the Inside Out*, Dr Libby expertly explains your outer world, the food you choose, the nutrients you ingest, hydration, posture, movement and what your body needs to create lovely nails, lustrous hair, sparkling eyes, and clear, luminous skin. Be guided to deal with very specific bumps in the road, such as dark circles under the eyes, eczema, pimples, and hair that is falling out, to name only a few. Just as importantly, Dr Libby explains your inner world, sex hormones, stress hormones, detox, digestion, elimination pathways, thyroid and pituitary functions. Both worlds relate to your sparkle. In addition taking a heart-opening look at your emotional landscape is important because, for many, that is where the real elixir is.

Beauty From The Inside Out is a must-have beauty bible for all women. Enjoy radiating your own unique sparkle, from the inside out. Dr Libby has also released an online course called Dr Libby's Essential Beauty Gems.